The Complete Ketogenic Diet
Cookbook for Beginners

*The Ultimate Keto Recipes
for Sustainable Weight Loss*

The Keto Academy of Italian Chefs

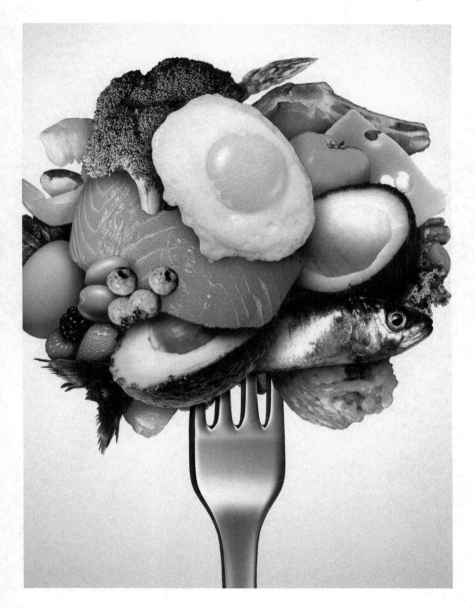

Table of Contents

INTRODUCTION **10**

THE KETO DIET AND THE RIGHT APPROACH 10

WHAT IS KETOSIS? 10

BUT WHAT'S ITS GOAL? 11

BENEFITS 12

CHAPTER 1 BREAKFAST **14**

KETO COFFEE 14

BULLETPROOF COFFEE 15

KETO BREAD 16

GRANNY'S BISCUITS 17

SWEETS BREAD ROLLS 18

MUSHROOMS OMELET 19

THUNDERING PLUMCAKE 20

CHEESE CRACKERS 21

FRUIT AND NUT CEREALS 22

QUEEN MUESLI 23

AL CAPONE CAPPUCCINO 24

SUPER WAFFLE 25

VEGAN COCONUT DONUTS 26

GALAXY PORRIDGE 27

SUPER MUFFIN 28

MOM'S BISCUITS 29

HOMEMADE KEFIR 30

DREAM BISCUITS 31

MOM'S COCONUT ROLLS 32

PROTEIN COCONUT PANCAKE 33

CHOCOLATE BISCUITS 34

MEDITERRANEAN FLATBREAD 35

COCONUT BISCUIT 36

IRONMAN PANCAKE 37

AMERICAN GYM COOKIE 38

TOAST BREAD 39

CHEDDAR BACON AND EGG FRITTATA 40

CINNAMON-CREAM-CHEESE ALMOND WAFFLES 41

ZUCCHINI AND CARROT COCONUT BREAD 42

CREAMY RICOTTA ALMOND CLOUD PANCAKES 43

CHAPTER 2 LUNCH AND DINNER **44**

ZUCCHINI SPAGHETTI WITH SHRIMPS 44

KING'S EGGS WITH AVOCADO 45

GNOCCHI – ITALIAN PASTA 46
BROCCOLI LASAGNA 47
MAJORETTE TUNA FILLET 48
VIVA ITALIA OMELETTE 49
SALT MUFFINS 50
PRINCE'S GRATINATED SCALLOPS... 51
RICOTTA AND SPINACH CRESPELLE 52
MEATLOAF... 54
CABBAGE AND LEMON SALAD 55
GREEK VEGETABLES 56
SANDWICH BREAD 57
KETO PIZZA 58
ZUCCHINI LASAGNA 59
IMPERIAL FLATBREAD... 60
SHRIMPS WITH SAUCE AND MERENGUE 61
PARMESAN EGGPLANT.. 62
HAM CHICKEN... 63
MUSHROOMS AND PARMESAN SALAD... 64
THE BARON'S COD 65
BEEF MEDALLIONS WITH ASPARAGUS.. 66
PARMESAN PIZZAS 67
AMERICAN PIZZA... 68
MINI ZUCCHINI HAMBURGER 69
FRIED SEABASS 70
ENGLISH BEEF.. 71
DELIVERY PIZZA 72
SESAME BUNS FOR HAMBURGERS... 73
KETO BREAD 74
CHICKEN FRIES.. 75
VEGETABLE FRIES 76
RUSSIAN SALAD WITH SALMON 77
THE PIRATE'S SWORDFISH 78
MEDITERRANEA HAKE 79
LEMON BREAM 80
CREAMY CHICKEN WITH GARLIC 81
SALMON ON CABBAGE 82
KING'S PORK CHOP 83
TUNA FILLET IN GREEN FIELDS 84
SPECK AND SALMON SKEWER 85
CHEESY MEATBALLS 86
SAUSAGE AND ONION PIE 87
SPINACH OMELET.. 88
TUNA AND EGGS SALAD 89

PIZZA 90
LIGHT RUSSIAN SALAD 91
QUEEN'S CAULIFLOWER SOUP 92
DANCING ZUCCHINI 93
BOLSHEVIK SHRIMPS 94
TUNA SAUCE 95
SOUTHERN ITALY SPICY CHICKEN 96
SQUASH BLOSSOMS IN LOVE 97
SUPER MAYO 98
CURRY CHICKEN 99
SALMON SOUP 100
LEMON CHICKEN 101
DELICIOUS BRIE 102
SEA MEATBALLS 103
DEVIL'S CHICKEN 104
ESKIMO SALMON 105
CHICKEN AND WALNUT STEWS 106
TUNA HAMBURGER 107
AVOCADO CRADLE 108
PARMESAN PIZZA 109
CHICKEN MUFFINS 110
GRANDPA'S GRILLED CHEESE 111
VIENNESE CHICKEN WINGS 112
FLOWERING MUSHROOMS 113
HOMEMADE CHEESE 114
CHEESE AND WALNUTS SALAD 115
SPIDERMAN SALAD 116
GENOVESE SQUIDS 117
TURMERIC FENNELS 118
SCOTTONA SLICES WITH PUMPKIN 119
EGGS WITH TUNA AND VEGGIES 120
CHORIZO, KALE, AND AVOCADO EGGS 121
DILL-CREAM-CHEESE SALMON ROLLS 122
CHEESE AND EGG SPINACH NESTS 123
MUSHROOM AND BROCCOLI QUICHE 124
TOMATO AND BACON CUPS 125
TRIPLE CHEESE AND BACON ZUCCHINI BALLS 126
PEPPERY OMELET WITH CHEDDAR CHEESE 127
AVOCADO SAUSAGE STACKS 129
MUSHROOM AND KALE TOFU SCRAMBLE 130
CREAM CHEESE ALMOND MUFFINS 131
SWISS CHARD, SAUSAGE, AND SQUASH OMELET 132
SAUSAGE QUICHE 133

GRUYERE AND MUSHROOM LETTUCE WRAPS 134

BACON AND ZUCCHINI HASH 135

FETA SPINACH FRITTATA 136

CHAPTER 3 SMOOTHIES **138**

CHOCOLATE SMOOTHIE IN THE WOODS 138

ST. CLAUS' SMOOTHIE 139

SUPERMAN SMOOTHIE 140

CHOCOLATE BOMB 141

WOOD PUDDING 142

FIT SMOOTHIE 143

HOT CHOCOLATE IN A CUP 144

SHAKED COLD COFFEE 145

BATMAN COCKTAIL 146

VEGETABLE SMOOTHIE 147

SUPERMAN SHAKE 148

ALMOND SHAKE 149

CHAPTER 4 DESSERT **150**

CHOCOLATE CAKE 150

BERRIES CHEESECAKE 151

MOM'S MASCARPONE 152

EXPLOSIVE CAKE 153

LEMON CAKE 154

DREAMY PANCAKES 155

LEMON PIE 156

COFFEE AND WALNUTS CAKE 157

ARTICHOKE HERBAL TEA 158

SUPERMAN'S SORBET 159

PARADISIAC ICE-CREAM 160

JAPANESE COTTON CHEESECAKE 161

VANILLA CAKE 162

COCONUT AND STRAWBERRIES SORBET 163

CHOCOLATE AND AVOCADO PUDDING 164

CHIA PUDDING 165

THE PRINCESS'S CAKE 166

INTRODUCTION

The ketogenic diet is not only a diet but a lifestyle. It's also about being aware of food, sustainable weight loss, and – mainly – improving and taking care of one's own body, even more so for people over 50.

The Keto Diet and the Right Approach

One of the main reasons why people suffer from obesity more and more often is that to lose weight, we have to cope with classical diets, which aren't sustainable and that one can't really follow in the long run. In fact, deciding to give up one's own alimentary habits, which are usually full of fat and sugar, is never easy to follow a diet based on privations. It will only take a lack of motivation or a simple problem, and the priority of losing weight will be put on the back burner, with the consequential interruption of the diet.

Add to this the fact that the temptations of sweets and carbohydrates are stronger than willpower because your brain is dependent on such foods. Assuming sugars or carbs create a hormonal disbalance that literally "drugs" your brain (there's a part of the brain called Nucleus Accumbens, where a certain idea of addiction is created, not only for what concerns sex or drugs but also sugars). According to this idea, the extent of the use of a certain substance determines precise transformations in the structures and functions of the brain, which transforms voluntary use in a compulsive search (Leshner, 1997). The evidence of this disease is the loss of control, enticing you towards these foods and pushing you to eat them continuously, in order to associate it with gratification, to the feeling of pleasure. Therefore, the most efficacious way to successfully change one's own diet is not giving up tasty products.

What is Ketosis?

Ketosis is a metabolic state characterized by the presence of ketones in the blood. This occurs when the body faces a "challenge" of low blood sugar levels and reduced glycogen stores, which initiates a cascade of hormones that signal the body to begin breaking down fat stores and releasing fatty acids into circulation. Once in circulation, these fatty acids are transported to the liver and used in ketone production. This process is called ketogenesis. To be more specific, the liver produces a ketone body known as acetoacetate (AcAc), most of which is converted into beta-hydroxybutyrate (BHB).

But What's Its Goal?

Most of us know that our bodies can produce energy by burning carbohydrates and fats. One of the main sources of energy for humans and animals is glucose, which is primarily obtained by consuming dietary carbohydrates: bread, fruits, vegetables, legumes, starches, and sugars.

Breaking down carbohydrates into glucose is one way to maintain blood sugar. Many tissues in the body use glucose as fuel and some can't use anything else (red blood cells, e.g.).

In addition to blood glucose, we can store glucose in our muscles and liver as glycogen, that is, long chains of glucose. We use glycogen during situations when blood glucose begins to decline, such as during long-duration exercise.

Humans can also burn fat for energy, and several organs - the heart, for example - prefer fat as their main energy substrate.

Fat: is also a great source of energy because we have plenty of it! Even the leanest among us have enough body fat to last us a long time.

The purpose of ketosis is to provide fuel when other energy sources (mainly glucose) are running low. This was the survival mechanism that allowed organisms to survive in conditions where the food supply was low. To keep energy levels high and maintain cognitive function, the liver produces ketones that serve as metabolic fuel for the brain and body.

Ketones, unlike fatty acids, can cross the blood-brain barrier that separates the brain from our circulation. This allows the brain to have a source of energy when glucose is low. During "starvation," up to 60% of the brain's energy may come from the body's ketone metabolism. Although ketosis isn't necessarily essential to "survive" in our modern world, this "unique" metabolic state surely has some benefits.

Benefits

Ketosis achieved through a ketogenic diet has been shown to have benefits for a wide variety of clinical conditions.

The keto diet originally began as a treatment for epilepsy and is still used in this way today. Ketone metabolism may have some powerful brain benefits, including reduced oxidative stress, lower inflammation levels, and improved levels of various neurotransmitters involved in health and disease processes.

The ketogenic diet has been shown to reduce seizure frequency in epilepsy patients by 40 to 90%.

Other brain conditions that benefit from ketosis include Alzheimer's disease and Parkinson's disease. There's also some evidence that ketosis may improve mood, reduce migraines, and increase mental focus.

Along with brain health, ketosis is effective in treating metabolic conditions such as type 2 diabetes, which is characterized by insulin resistance. The keto diet reduces blood sugar and lipids, increases weight loss, and improves insulin sensitivity, which reduces the risk of diabetes and metabolic syndrome or mitigates its negative effects.

The metabolic benefits of keto could extend to athletes since ketosis is characterized by the possibility to burn fat.

Several studies have shown that athletes who follow a keto diet can significantly improve their body composition: building lean muscle mass while reducing body fat.

Ketosis can be achieved endogenously (using exercise, fasting or a **ketogenic diet**) or exogenously using exogenous ketone supplements. Many benefits of ketosis are similar, regardless of the method obtained to induce it. However, these benefits are particularly related to weight and fat loss.

We wish you a "good keto"! Take care!

Chapter 1
Breakfast

Keto Coffee

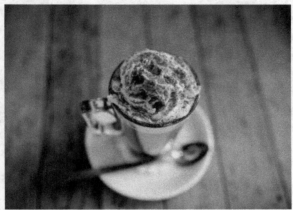

Ingredients for 1 portion:
- 1 Espresso (also mocha coffee is fine)
- ½ teaspoon of ground cinnamon
- 1 cup water
- ¼ cup of unsweetened whipping cream

Nutrition 100 g:
Calories: 136 kcal
Fat: 10 g
Proteins: 1 g
Carbs: 1 g
Directions:
1. Prepare your espresso (you can also do it with a mocha).
2. Add hot water.
3. Serve coffee in a longer cup and add some whipping cream on top.
4. Sprinkle some ground cinnamon.
Enjoy the beginning of your day!

Bulletproof Coffee

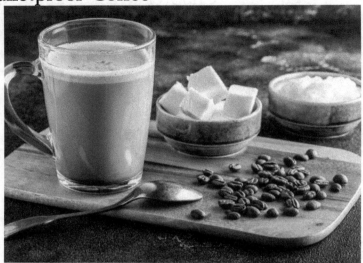

Ingredients for 1 portion:
- 1 tall espresso or mocha coffee
- 1 tsp ghee or clarified butter
- 1 tsp of coconut oil
- Stevia or erythritol to taste

Nutrition 100 g:
Calories: 144 kcal
Fat: 16 g
Proteins: 0 g
Carbs: 0 g

Directions:
1. Brew your espresso or mocha coffee.
2. Add 1 tsp butter and coconut oil.
3. Pour it in a cup while hot and whisk.
4. If you prefer, sweeten it with stevia or erythritol.
You'll rock it!

Keto Bread

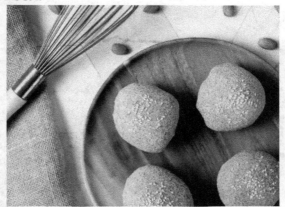

Ingredients for 4 portions/rolls:
- 1 cup almond flour
- ½ tsp psyllium powder
- ¾ cup water
- 4 small egg whites
- 1 tsp apple cider vinegar
- Extra virgin olive oil to taste
- Baking powder q.s.
- Salt to taste

Nutrition 100 g:
Calories: 220 kcal
Fat: 20 g
Proteins: 14 g
Carbs: 5 g
Directions:
1. Preheat your oven at 350° F.
2. Mix the dry ingredients in a bowl and boil water.
3. Add vinegar and egg whites to dry ingredients and mix.
4. Add boiled water and whisk for about 30 seconds until it reaches a chewy consistency.
5. Moisten your hands with a little bit of oil and shape the dough.
6. Put it on a baking plate lined with parchment paper.
7. Bake on the lower rack of the oven for 50-60 minutes.
Enjoy!

Granny's Biscuits

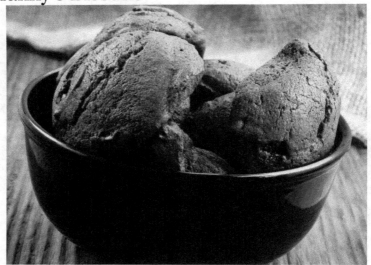

Ingredients for 10 biscuits:

- ¾ almond flour
- 1/4 cup ghee or clarified butter
- 3 and ¾ cups coconut flour
- 70 gr egg whites
- ¼ cup erythritol
- 2 tbsp of cocoa powder
- 1 tsp xanthan

Nutrition 100 g:

Calories: 504 kcal

Fat: 28 g

Proteins: 18 g

Carbs: 5 g

Directions:

1. Combine all the dry ingredients in a bowl.

2. Add egg whites and butter and whisk until you get an elastic and homogeneous dough.

3. Shape the dough as you wish.

4. Cook for 20 minutes at 320° F.

The classical Italian breakfast!

Sweets Bread Rolls

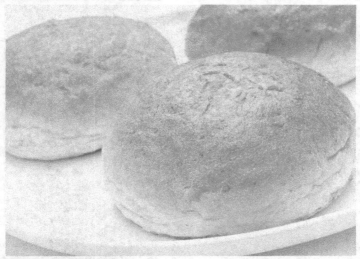

Ingredients for 3-4 rolls:
- ¼ cup of linseed flour
- ¾ tbsp of coconut flour
- ¼ tbsp of xanthan powder
- 1 tbsp erythritol
- 1/4 cups clarified butter
- 3 eggs

Nutrition 100 g:
Calories: 544 kcal
Fat: 30 g
Proteins: 22 g
Carbs: 4 g

Directions:
1. Mix eggs and erythritol in a bowl.
2. Combine the different types of flour with your hands until you get an elastic and homogeneous dough.
3. Divide the dough into 3-4 balls.
4. Cook for 30 minutes at 350° F.
Everybody loves sweet bread rolls!

Mushrooms Omelet

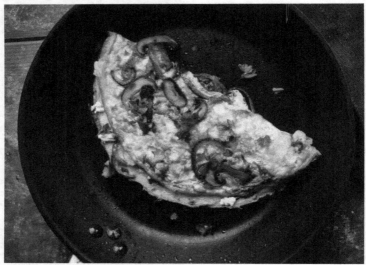

Ingredients for 1 portion:

- 2 sliced mushrooms
- 2 eggs
- ¼ cup grated cheese
- 1 and ½ clarified butter
- 1/4 onion, finely chopped
- Salt, pepper and parsley to taste

Nutrition 100 g:
Calories: 240 kcal
Fat: 24 g
Proteins: 20 g
Carbs: 3 g
Directions:
1. In a bowl, beat the eggs and add a pinch of salt and pepper.
2. Heat a skillet and melt butter, sauteing onions and mushrooms until tender.
3. Pour eggs on mushrooms and onions to cover.
4. When the omelet begins to firm up, sprinkle with cheese.
5. Continue cooking until it's formed.
Here you go!

Thundering Plumcake

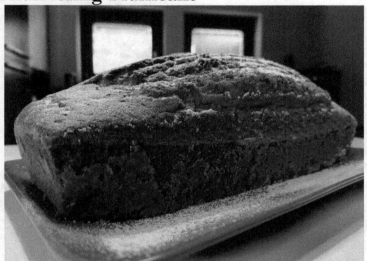

Ingredients for 6-8 people:

- 3 eggs
- ½ cup Evo oil
- 2 cups almond flour
- 1 cup coconut flour
- 80 g erythritol
- ¾ cup white yogurt
- 1 tsp of baking soda
- Juice of ½ lemon

Nutrition 100 g:
Calories: 340 kcal
Fat: 24 g
Proteins: 18 g
Carbs: 5 g
Directions:
1. Whisk eggs with erythritol, yogurt, oil, baking soda and lemon juice.
2. Gradually add the two types of flour and mix well.
3. Pour the mixture into a buttered plum cake mold.
4. Cook for 30 minutes at 400° F.
Here you've got some thunders!

Cheese Crackers

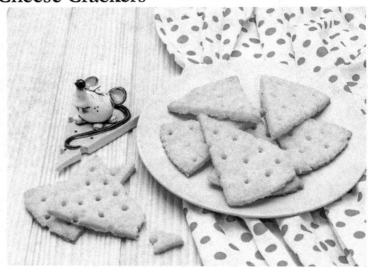

Ingredients for 4 portions:

- Salt
- Rosemary
- 1 egg
- ¼ cup cream cheese
- 2 cups grated cheese
- 1 cup almond flour

Nutrition 100 g:
Calories: 580 kcal
Fat: 27 g
Proteins: 18 g
Carbs: 5 g
Directions:

1. First of all, get a mixer (or do it by hand) and pour inside all the ingredients. Mix until you get a homogeneous mix.
2. Put the mixture on some baking paper placed on a baking sheet. Take another baking paper and cover the mixture.
3. Use a rolling pin to roll the dough out until it reaches a 1cm thickness.
4. At this point, cut the dough into small pieces with a knife. Put the pan in the oven and cook for some minutes at 400° F until they're brown.

Aren't they crispy?!

Fruit and Nut Cereals

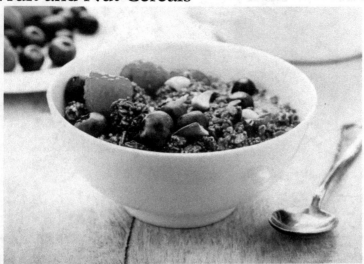

Ingredients for 1 portion:
- 2 tbsp berries
- 2 tbsp almonds
- 2 tbsp walnuts
- 2 tbsp oats
- 2 tbsp erythritol
- 1 tbsp coconut milk

Nutrition 100 g:
Calories: 308 kcal
Carbs: 5 g
Proteins: 14 g
Fat: 30 g
Directions:
1. Combine fruits and cereals in a bowl.
2. Add coconut milk and mix.
Here you got wellness-made food!

Queen Muesli

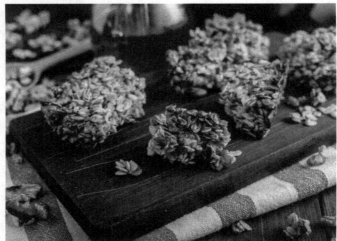

Ingredients for 3 portions:

- 1 cup coconut flakes
- 1 cup sunflower seeds
- 1 cup pumpkin seeds
- 1 cup chopped almonds
- 1/2 cup walnuts
- 1/2 cup hemp seeds
- 2 teaspoons cinnamon
- 1/2 teaspoon vanilla extract
- 1 tablespoon of Erythritol

Later on:

- Almond milk without sugar to taste

Nutrition 100 g:

Calories: 310 kcal

Carbs: 7 g

Proteins: 15 g

Fat: 36 g

Directions:

1. Mix all the ingredients and put the resulting mixture in a baking dish.

2. Bake in the oven at 360° for about 7-8 minutes. Let it cool.

3. Serve with almond milk.

Superfine!

Al Capone Cappuccino

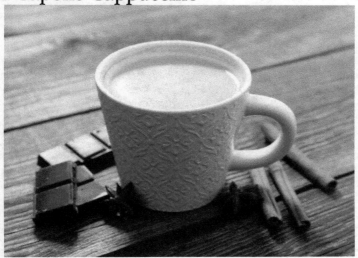

Ingredients for 1 portion:
- 1/4 cup coconut milk
- 1 tbsp bitter cocoa powder
- 1 tbsp erythritol
- 1 tbsp vanilla
- ¾ cup unsweetened almond milk
- 1 tbsp coconut oil

Nutrition 100 g:
Calories: 270 kcal
Carbs: 5 g
Proteins: 9 g
Fat: 18 g
Directions:
1. Place all the ingredients in a pot. Simmer everything for 8 minutes, stirring occasionally.
2. Let it cool and then pour your Cappuccino in a cup.
Good morning with a miter!

Super Waffle

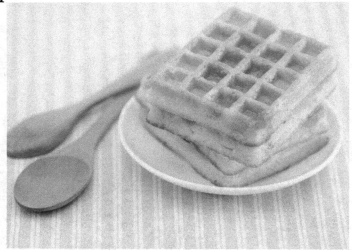

Ingredients for 3 portions:
- 4 eggs
- 4 tbsp coconut oil
- 1 and ¼ coconut milk
- 1 tbsp baking powder
- 3 egg whites
- 1 and ½ almond flour

Nutrition 100 g:
Calories: 487 kcal
Carbs: 9 g
Proteins: 24 g
Fat: 38 g
Directions:
1.Preheat the waffle iron.
2. Combine all the dry ingredients in a bowl. Add the liquid ones gradually, mix well and let the mixture rest for 5 minutes.
3. Pour everything into the waffle iron and cook for a few minutes. You'll feel like Superman!

Vegan Coconut Donuts

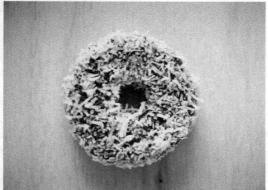

Ingredients for 3 portions:
- ¾ cup almond flour
- ¼ cup coconut flour
- 1 tbsp xanthan powder
- 3 eggs
- 1/2 tsp baking soda
- 1/2 tsp baking powder
- 1/2 tsp coffee
- 1/3 cup unsweetened almond milk
- 1 tbsp of Erythritol
- 3 tbsp unsweetened cocoa powder
- 1/4 cup coconut oil
- 1 tbsp coconut flakes

Nutrition 100 g:
Calories: 362 kcal **Carbs:** 7 g
Proteins: 12 g **Fat:** 28 g
Directions:
1. Preheat your oven at 360° F.
2. Grease a baking pan and put it aside.
3. Add all the ingredients in a bowl and mix until they're homogeneously mixed.
4. Pour the mixture into the pan and put it in the oven for 20 minutes.
5. Sprinkle with coconut flakes (optional)
Here you go! Your American breakfast!

Galaxy Porridge

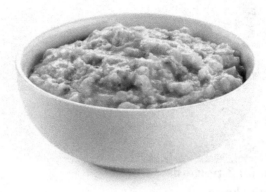

Ingredients for 1 portion:
- ¼ almond flour
- 1/2 tsp cinnamon
- 3 tsp vanilla extract
- 1 tsp erythritol
- 1 tbsp chia seeds
- 2 tbsp of ground flax seed
- ½ cup of hemp seeds
- 1 cup unsweetened almond milk

Nutrition for 1 portion:
Calories: 367 kcal
Carbs: 7 g
Proteins: 18 g
Fat: 29 g

Directions:
1. Add all the ingredients in a pot and mix well.
2. Cook over medium heat, mix and cook until it boils and 2 minutes more.

An English classic!

Super Muffin

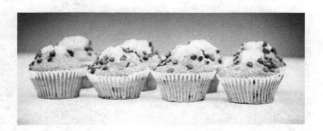

Ingredients for 8/10 Muffins:
- 3 eggs
- ½ cup almond flour
- ½ cup erythritol
- ¼ butter
- 40 gr dark chocolate flakes
- ¼ tsp salt
- 1 tsp baking powder

Nutrition 100 g:
Calories: 319 kcal
Fat: 30 g
Proteins: 7 g
Carbs: 6 g
Directions:
1. Beat the eggs with the whips.
2. Gradually add the coconut flour and erythritol and mix well.
3. Add melted butter and then all the other ingredients.
4. Pour the mixture into the muffin molds and bake in a preheated oven at 360° F for 20 minutes.
That's what we call a breakfast!

Mom's Biscuits

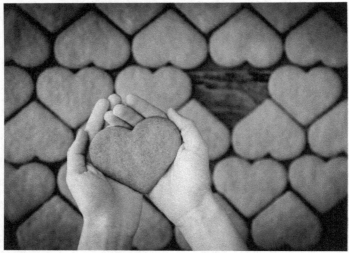

Ingredients:

- ¼ cup coconut oil
- 30 gr erythritol
- ¾ cup almond flour
- 1 egg
- 1 tsp of tartar cream
- 1 tsp of baking soda

Nutrition 100 g:

Carbs: 7 g
Proteins: 20 g
Fat: 50 g
Calories: 132 kcal

Directions:

1. Mix all ingredients in a bowl, form a dough, and wrap it in plastic wrap, let it rest in the refrigerator for an hour.

2. Roll out the dough on baking paper and cut out cookie shapes half an inch thick.

3. Bake at 360° F until they're brown.

You'll lose your mind!

Homemade Kefir

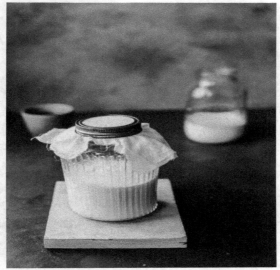

Kefir gives innumerable and essential benefits. Here's why we're suggesting you how to do it and to assume it before breakfast:

Ingredients 1, 1 liter:

- 100 gr Kefir milk
- 1000 gr Fresh milk

Nutrition 100 g:

Calories: 74 kcal

Fat: 5 g

Proteins: 4 g

Carbs: 3 g

Directions:

1. Premise: for every 100 gr of milk, you need 10 gr of Kefir (10%).

2. Put 100 gr of Kefir milk in a large glass cup with a lid and add fresh milk gradually, mixing with a plastic or wooden spoon (don't ever use a metal one!).

3. Cover it with a clean cotton cloth and close it with an elastic band.

4. Leave the container indoors without light to ferment for at least 12 hours. You can go up to 24 hours if you want it thicker and to make sure the lactose has disappeared, giving space to the lactic ferments.

5. Store it in the refrigerator.

It'll be creamy and tasty!

Dream Biscuits

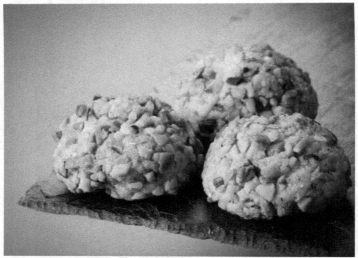

Ingredients:
- 5 tbsp walnuts, chopped
- 5 tbsp chopped pistachios
- 5 tbsp almond grains
- 2 egg yolks
- 1 tbsp butter
- 1 tbsp mascarpone cheese

Nutrition 100 g:
Calories: 474 kcal
Fat: 35 g
Proteins: 30 g
Carbs: 7 g
Directions:
1. Combine walnuts, pistachios, and almond grains.
2. Combine yolks with butter and mascarpone cheese in a bowl.
3. Combine the two mixtures and mix, shape balls and make them on a baking sheet lined with parchment paper.
4. Bake for 10-15 minutes at 340° F.
5. Sprinkle with dark cacao or dark chocolate flakes.
You'll close your eyes once you taste them!

Mom's Coconut Rolls

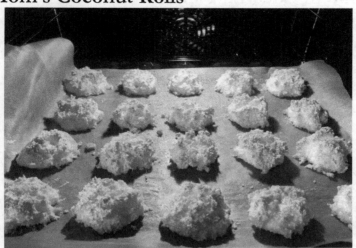

Ingredients:
- ½ cups + 2 tbsp almond flour
- ½ coconut, chopped
- 1 cup egg whites
- 30 gr erythritol

Nutrition 100 g:
Calories: 494 kcal
Fat: 42 g
Proteins: 30 g
Carbs: 5 g

Directions:
1. Whip the egg whites well, then add the other ingredients and mix, preferably by hand.
2. Bake in a static oven at 340° F for 10-15 minutes.
Mamma mia!

Protein Coconut Pancake

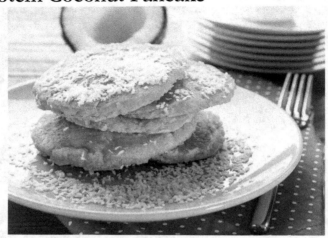

Ingredients:

- 1 egg
- 1 tbsp erythritol
- 2 tbsp coconut flour
- 2 tbsp almond flour
- 50 g almond milk without added sugar
- 1 tbsp milk protein powder
- 1 tsp baking powder

Nutrition 100 g:

Calories: 340 kcal

Fat: 24 g

Proteins: 22 g

Carbs: 5 g

Directions:

1. In a medium-sized bowl, combine the powdered ingredients (flours, proteins, baking powder, sweetener) and mix everything together. At this point, add eggs and mix, and then pour in the milk while stirring continuously.

2. When the mixture is homogeneous, pour a part of it in the center of the non-stick pan, which you will have heated on medium heat, cook 2-3 minutes, and turn (if it has made bubbles, it means that it's ready to turn), cook the other side and serve. You can sprinkle it with whatever you like.

The classical Dessert!

Chocolate Biscuits

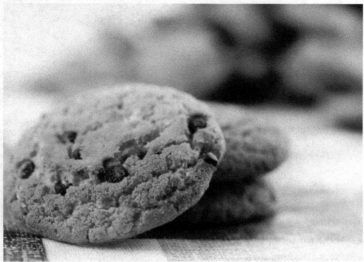

Ingredients:

- 1 cup almond flour
- 1 cup coconut flour
- ¼ butter
- 2 eggs
- 30 gr erythritol
- 50 dark chocolate flakes
- Salt to taste

Nutrition 100 g:
Calories: 491 kcal
Fat: 40 g
Proteins: 30 g
Carbs: 5 g
Directions:
1. Mix together the two flours in a bowl, then pour and swirl in the melted butter.
2. Add the two eggs and the sweetener and mix well.
3. When the dough is smooth, take 4/5 chocolate chips at a time and, together with the dough, make little balls.
4. Bake at 380° F for 15-20 minutes.
These cookies will make you dream!

Mediterranean Flatbread

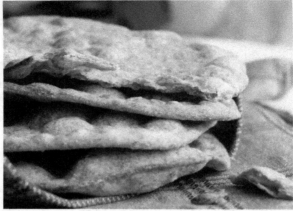

Ingredients:

- ½ cup coconut flour
- 1 tbsp psyllium husk powder
- ¼ cup olive oil - 1 cup boiling water
- ½ cup grated parmesan or mozzarella cheese
- ½ tsp salt - ¼ tsp grated garlic
- ½ tsp pepper
- ½ tbsp dried rosemary

Nutrition 100 g:
Calories: 621 kcal **Fat:** 54 g **Proteins:** 24 g **Carbs:** 10 g
Directions:
1. Whisk the dry ingredients (flour, psyllium, salt, garlic, pepper, and rosemary) together in a bowl.
2. Add olive oil and cheese.
3. Add hot water, stirring.
4. Continue stirring until the psyllium fiber and coconut flour have absorbed all the water.
5. Flatten the dough on baking paper on a baking sheet.
6. Roll or press the dough until it's thin and even. Make sure it's a thickness of less than ⅛ inch.
7. Bake at 360° F for 20-25 minutes (baking time depends on the thickness of the dough).
8. After browning, transfer to a cooling rack, remove the baking paper and let the focaccia cool. Try it with some salami or prosciutto, you'll go crazy!

Coconut Biscuit

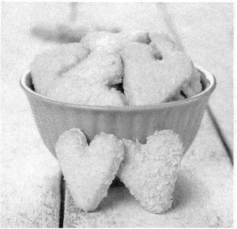

Ingredients 1 biscuit:

- 1 tbsp coconut flour
- 1 tsp coconut, grated and dehydrated
- 1 egg white
- ½ tsp coconut oil
- 1 tsp cinnamon
- ½ tsp vanilla aroma

Nutrition 100 g:
Calories: 593 kcal
Fat: 50 g
Proteins: 22 g
Carbs: 5 g

Directions:

1. Whip the egg whites together with the vanilla, add the coconut flour, coconut oil, grated coconut and mix until smooth.

2. Roll out on a flat surface and cut out cookies.

3. Sprinkle with more coconut flakes and bake at 320° F for about 20 minutes.

Eat them warm and you'll taste paradise!

Ironman Pancake

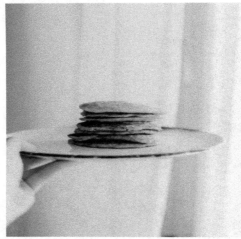

Ingredients for 1 portion:
- ¼ cup lupin flour
- ½ cup whipped oat flakes, reduced to flour
- 1 cup egg white
- 5 gr erythritol
- ¼ vanilla powder to taste

Nutrition 100 g:
Calories: 502 kcal
Fat: 40 g
Proteins: 22 g
Carbs: 7 g

Directions:
1. Place all the ingredients in a bowl and mix with your hands until you get a well-blended dough.
2. Shape balls and use baking paper underneath and on top by pressing them with a rolling pin until circles are made.
3. Bake in a skillet with coconut oil until firm.
4. You can garnish with anything you like.
That's the real American breakfast!

American Gym Cookie

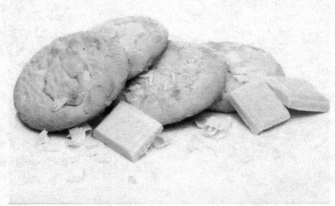

Ingredients for 4 biscuits:

- ¼ cup almond flour
- ¼ cup lupin flour
- 1/4 cup protein powder
- 1 tsp dark cocoa
- ½ cup egg white
- 1 tbsp white chocolate, cubed
- 1 tsp erythritol

Nutrition:
Calories: 268 kcal
Carbs: 5 g
Proteins: 34 g
Fat: 12 g
Directions:
1. Heat your oven at 360° F.
2. Prepare a bowl and pour almond and lupin flour, erythritol, cocoa and start mixing.
3. Add egg whites and keep on mixing until you get a soft and homogeneous mixture.
4. Divide the dough, shape 4 biscuits and put them on a pan (don't forget baking paper).
5. Sprinkle white chocolate on them.
6. Cook for 10 minutes at 360° F.
You'll feel renewed!

Toast Bread

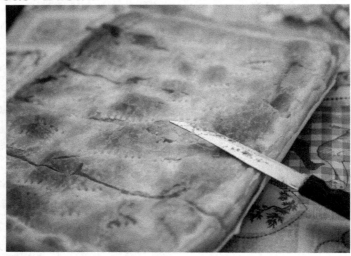

Ingredients:
- 1 cup egg whites
- Oregano or Rosemary
- salt to taste

Nutrition 100 g:
Calories: 68 kcal
Carbs: 1 g
Proteins: 10 g
Fat: 1 g

Directions:
1. Pour egg whites in a bowl with salt, oregano and beat with a mixer.
2. Prepare a pan and place some baking paper on it (35 x 25), pour the mixture on the pan and season with more oregano or rosemary.
3. Bake for 20 minutes at 400° F.
4. Divide among plates to get 3 toasts.
Enjoy!

Cheddar Bacon and Egg Frittata

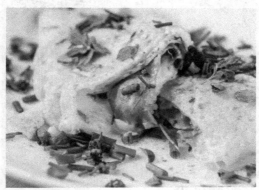

Ingredients for 4 portions:

- 8 slices bacon
- 8 fresh eggs
- 4 tablespoons butter ghee, melted
- ½ cup almond milk, possibly lactose-free
- Salt and black pepper to taste
- 2 cups Cheddar cheese, shredded
- ¼ cup chopped green onions
- ¼ cup Greek yogurt

Nutritional values 1 person:
Calories: 326 Kcal **Fat:** 28 g
Protein: 15 g
Carbs: 2 g
Directions:
1. Preheat the oven to 400°F (205°C) and grease a baking dish with cooking spray.
2. Cook the bacon in a skillet over medium heat for 6 minutes. Once crispy, remove from the skillet to paper towels and discard grease. Chop into small pieces.
3. Whisk the eggs, butter, milk, salt, and black pepper.
4. Mix in the bacon and pour the mixture into the baking dish. Sprinkle with Cheddar cheese and green onions, and bake in the oven for 10 minutes or until the eggs are thoroughly cooked.
5. Remove and cool the frittata for 3 minutes, slice into wedges, and serve warm with a dollop of Greek yogurt.

Cinnamon-Cream-Cheese Almond Waffles

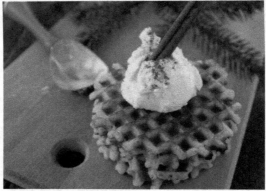

Ingredients for 6 portions:
Spread:

- 8 ounces (230g) cream cheese, at room temperature
- 1 teaspoon cinnamon powder - 3 tablespoons of erythritol
- Cinnamon powder for garnishing

Waffles:

- 5 tablespoons melted butter
- 1½ cups unsweetened almond milk
- 8 eggs - ¼ teaspoon liquid stevia
- ½ teaspoon baking powder - 2 cups almond flour

Nutritional values:
Calories: 308 Kcal **Fat:** 24 g **Protein:** 12 g **Carbs:** 8 g
Directions:
1. Combine the cream cheese, cinnamon, and erythritol with a hand mixer until smooth.
2. To make the waffles, whisk the butter, milk, and eggs in a medium bowl. Add the stevia and baking powder and mix.
3. Stir in the almond flour and combine until no lumps exist. Let the batter sit for 5 minutes to thicken.
4. Spritz a waffle iron with a non-stick cooking spray.
5. Ladle a ¼ cup of the batter into the waffle iron and cook until golden, about 10 minutes in total. Repeat with the remaining batter.
6. Slice the waffles into quarters; apply the cinnamon spread in between each of two waffles and snap. Sprinkle with cinnamon powder and serve.

Zucchini and Carrot Coconut Bread

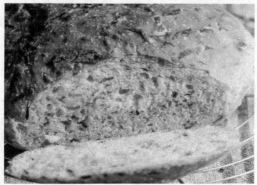

Ingredients for 4 portions:
- 1 cup shredded carrots
- 1 cup shredded zucchini, squeezed
- ½ cup coconut flour
- 1 teaspoon vanilla extract
- 6 eggs
- 1 tablespoon coconut oil
- ¾ teaspoon baking soda
- 1 tablespoon cinnamon powder
- ½ teaspoon salt
- ½ cup Greek yogurt
- 1 teaspoon apple cider vinegar
- ½ teaspoon nutmeg powder

Nutritional values:
Calories: 177 Kcal **Fat:** 10 g **Protein:** 12 g **Carbs:** 2 g
Directions:
1.Preheat the oven to 350°F (180°C) and grease the loaf pan with cooking spray. Set aside.
2. Mix the carrots, zucchini, coconut flour, vanilla extract, eggs, coconut oil, baking soda, cinnamon powder, salt, Greek yogurt, vinegar, and nutmeg.
3. Pour the batter into the loaf pan and bake for 55 minutes.
4. Remove the bread after and let cool for 5 minutes.
5. Preserve the bread and use it for toasts, sandwiches, or served with soups and salads.

Creamy Ricotta Almond Cloud Pancakes

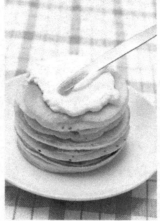

Ingredients for 4 portions:
- 1 cup almond flour 1 teaspoon baking powder
- 2½ tablespoons Swerve
- ⅓ teaspoon salt
- 1¼ cups ricotta cheese
- ⅓ cup coconut milk
- 2 large eggs
- 1 cup heavy whipping cream

Nutritional values:
Calories: 406 Kcal **Fat:** 30 g **Protein:** 11 g **Carbs:** 6 g

Directions:
1. In a medium bowl, whisk the almond flour, baking powder, Swerve, and salt. Set aside.
2. Crack the eggs into the blender and process on medium speed for 30 seconds.
3. Add the ricotta cheese, continue processing it, and gradually pour the coconut milk in while you keep on blending. In about 90 seconds, the mixture will be creamy and smooth.
4. Pour it into the dry ingredients and whisk to combine.
5. Set a skillet over medium heat and let it heat for a minute.
6. Then, fetch a soup spoonful of mixture into the skillet and cook it for 1 minute. Flip the pancake and cook further for 1 minute.
7. Remove onto a plate and repeat the cooking process until the batter is exhausted. Serve the pancakes with whipping cream.

Chapter 2
Lunch and Dinner

Zucchini Spaghetti with Shrimps

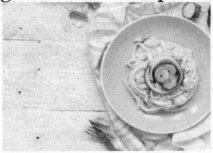

Ingredients for 1 portion:
- 1 and ¼ cups zucchini
- ½ cup shrimps
- ½ lactose-free cooking cream
- 1 tbsp mayo
- ¼ cup grated cheese
- ½ tbsp ghee or clarified butter

Nutrition 100 g:
Calories: 270 kcal
Fat: 22 g
Proteins: 23 g
Carbs: 3 g
Directions:
1. Heat the cooking cream in a pan, bring it to a boil and reduce slightly. Heat butter in another skillet and cook shrimps until brown; set aside. Add the cream and turn off the heat.

2. Wash the zucchini and cut them into thin strips with a potato peeler (or the appropriate tool). Cook the zucchini spaghetti for 30 seconds in a pot of boiling water. Add the cooking cream and shrimps, stirring to combine. Add grated cheese and serve.

Go Italian!

King's Eggs with Avocado

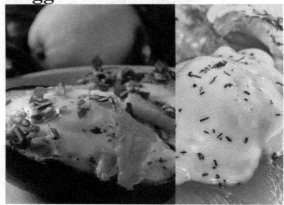

Ingredients 1 portion:
For the sauce:
- 1 egg yolk
- 1 tsp lemon juice
- ¼ cup ghee or clarified butter
- Salt and pepper to taste

For the King's Eggs:
- 1 avocado - 1 egg
- 40 gr smoked salmon

Nutrition 100 g:
Calories: 407 kcal **Fat:** 47 g **Proteins:** 16 g **Carbs:** 3 g

Directions:
1. Combine the egg yolk, lemon juice and butter and blend until a creamy white mixture forms. Season with salt and pepper to taste.
2. Put a saucepan with a little water on the stove and bring to boil, then reduce the heat.
3. Crack the egg and then gently slide it into the water. Stir the water around the egg.
4. Cook for 3 to 4 minutes, depending on your preference. Remove the poached egg from the water, helping with a scoop or place it on a paper towel to absorb excess water.
5. Cut the avocado in half and remove the stone and peel. Cut a slice at the base of each half so that it rests evenly on the plate.
6. Top the two halves first with the salmon and then with the egg and add a generous spoonful of hollandaise sauce. You'll feel like a King!

Gnocchi – Italian Pasta

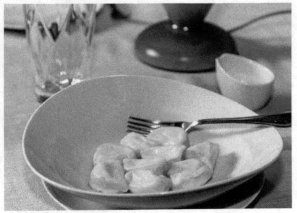

Ingredients for 4 portions:

- 1 cup almond flour
- 1/2 cup coconut flour
- ¾ grated parmesan cheese
- ¼ cup ricotta cheese
- 4 eggs
- 2 garlic cloves, chopped
- ½ cup butter
- 1 tbsp xanthan gum powder
- 4 tsp extra virgin olive oil
- Salt to taste

Nutrition 100 g:

Calories: 311 kcal **Fat:** 29 g **Proteins:** 12 g **Carbs:** 7 g

Directions:

1. Mix the almond flour with coconut flour and xanthan gum.
2. In a separate bowl, beat the egg and combine with ricotta, salt, and parmesan, mixing until smooth.
3. Add the cheese mixture to the flour mixture and mix well until it becomes a sticky ball.
4. Wrap the dough ball in plastic wrap and let it rest in the refrigerator for one hour. Shape the dough into small dumplings.
6. In a skillet, heat the olive oil and butter. Sauté the crushed garlic.
7. Pour the gnocchi into the skillet and cook for 5 to 6 minutes.
Enjoy!

Broccoli Lasagna

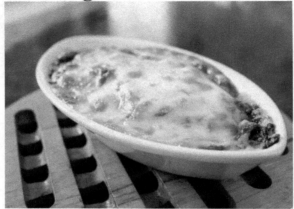

Ingredients for 4 portions:
- 1 cup broccoli
- ½ cup fresh spinach
- ½ cup shallot
- ½ cup butter
- 12 eggs
- 1 cup goat cheese
- 1 cup leafy vegetables
- 4 tbsp oil
- Salt and pepper to taste

Nutrition 100 g:
Calories: 477 kcal **Fat:** 67 g
Proteins: 35 g **Carbs:** 6 g
Directions:
1. Preheat the oven at 350° F.
2. Crack the eggs into a bowl and beat them with a whisk.
3. Grate or crumble the cheese and add it to the mixture.
4. Add salt and pepper to taste.
5. Chop broccoli and mince shallot.
6. Melt the butter in a skillet and cook broccoli and shallot over medium heat for 15 minutes. Add spinach to the pan and sauté for 1-2 minutes..Pour the vegetables into a baking dish and pour in the egg mixture. Place in the oven and bake for about 20 minutes. Mamma mia!

Majorette Tuna Fillet

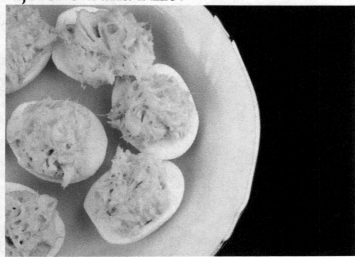

Ingredients 1 portion:

- 2 eggs
- 1 cup tuna fillet
- 1 tbsp mayo
- 1/2 onion
- Salt and pepper to taste

Nutrition 100 g:
Calories: 275 kcal
Fat: 29 g
Proteins: 26 g
Carbs: 1 g
Directions:
1. Bring a pot of water to a boil and pour the eggs in, letting them cook for 8 minutes.
2. In a bowl, mix the tuna fillet, mayonnaise, onion, salt, and pepper. Cut the hard-boiled eggs in half and place them on a plate and place the tuna mixture on top of the eggs.
Mouthwatering!

Viva Italia Omelette

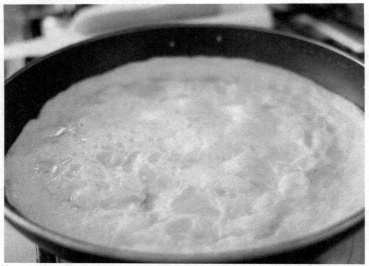

Ingredients for 2 portions:
- 4 egg whites
- ¼ butter
- ½ cup grated parmesan cheese
- Salt and pepper to taste – or any other spice

Nutrition 100 g:
Calories: 215 kcal
Fat: 29 g
Proteins: 25 g
Carbs: 0 g

Directions:
1. Pour the four egg whites into a glass cruet, beat well with a whisk while adding salt and spices.
2. Heat the butter in a pan until melted, then add the four beaten egg whites and close with a lid, turning occasionally.
3. As soon as it begins to solidify, add the parmesan cheese evenly on top. It will be ready in a heartbeat!
Get ready guys, it's delicious!
You may ask yourself what to do with the four yolks!
Well, let's not throw anything away, let's make "Mom's Mascarpone". (Go find it among the desserts)

Salt Muffins

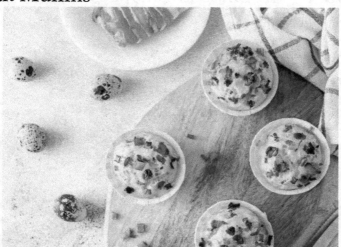

Ingredients 1 portion:
- 2 eggs
- 1 tbsp grated cheddar cheese
- 1 tbsp diced bacon
- 1/4 onion, finely chopped
- Salt and pepper to taste

Nutrition:
Calories: 266 kcal
Fat: 21 g
Proteins: 16 g
Carbs: 2 g
Directions:
1. Heat oven to 350° F and grease – with butter - two muffin molds.
2. Add the onion and bacon to the bottom of each mold.
3. In a bowl, beat the eggs with cheese and add the salt and pepper.
4. Pour the mixture into the two molds and bake the muffins in the oven for 20 minutes until firm.
Cheers!

Prince's Gratinated Scallops

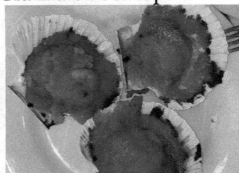

Ingredients for 1 portion:
- 3 whole scallops
- ½ cup shrimps
- salt, pepper, garlic, and parsley to taste
- 1 tbsp lemon juice
- ¼ cup breadcrumbs (low carb, if possible)

For the Light Béchamel:
- ¼ cup lupin flour
- ¼ olive oil
- 1 and ¼ milk
- 1 pinch nutmeg, salt and pepper

Nutrition:
Calories: 70 kcal **Carbs:** 5 g **Proteins:** 6 g **Fat:** 10 g

Directions:
1. Let the scallops open by placing them in a pot on the stove. When they've hatched, open with the help of a knife and free them from the fruit. Discard the black part, keep the rest.

2. Wash the shells well. Prepare the béchamel sauce: Place the flour in a saucepan, add the oil, begin to stir over low heat, add the milk little by little while stirring until it thickens. Ready. Cook shrimps in water and let cool. Cut scallops and shrimp into small pieces and add to béchamel sauce along with garlic, lemon juice, salt, pepper, and parsley. Fill scallop shells, then sprinkle with breadcrumbs.

3. Line a baking sheet with parchment paper, place the scallops with a drizzle of oil on top.

8. Bake for about 15 minutes in a preheated oven at 400° F.

Taste the divine!

Ricotta and Spinach Crespelle

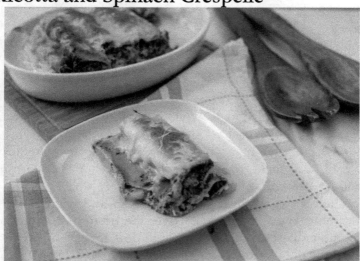

Ingredients:
For the Crespelle:

- 1 egg
- ½ cup egg white
- ¾ unsweetened milk
- 1 cup flour (oat or lupin flour)

For the Ricotta and Spinach filling:

- 150 g ricotta
- ½ cup spinach*
- 1 tsp parmesan
- 1 pinch fresh basil
- Salt and pepper to taste

For the Light Béchamel:

- ¼ cup lupin flour
- ¼ cup Evo oil
- 1 and ¼ milk (better without lactose)
- 1 pinch nutmeg, salt and pepper

Suggestions:

- 3 slices light cheese
- 2 tbsp tomato sauce
- 1 tbsp parmesan

Nutrition for 1 crespelle:
Calories: 220 kcal
Carbs: 9 g
Proteins: 21 g
Fat: 14 g
Directions:
For the Crespelle:
1. Prepare the crepes dough, while it rests, prepare the béchamel sauce, and cook the spinach.
2. In a bowl, combine eggs with the egg white, beating with a fork or whisk. Add flour milk gradually, combining well. Cover with plastic wrap and let stand 30'.
3. Once time's passed, heat a non-stick pan and when it becomes very hot, pour enough dough to cover the bottom. As soon as the edges come away, turn and cook a little less than 1', continue with the rest of the dough until done.
4. There should be 7 in all.

For the Light Béchamel:
- Place the flour in a saucepan, add oil, begin to stir over low heat, slowly add the milk while continuing to stir until it becomes thick. It's ready.

For the Ricotta and Spinach Filling:
1. Cook spinach in a skillet without adding anything else, and once hot, drain it.
2. Blend it together with ricotta, basil, parmesan, 2 tablespoons of béchamel, salt and pepper and set aside.

Now put it all together:
1. On the bottom of the baking dish, put 2 tablespoons of bechamel sauce and distribute well (to prevent the crepes from sticking).
2. Take a crepe and put a generous spoonful of filling on one side.
3. Cut the cheese slices into strips and place as many as you need on top of the filling.
4. Roll up the crepe, continue until you run out of ingredients, then place the crepes in a baking dish.
5. Pour the remaining béchamel over the crepes, finish by sprinkling 10 g of Parmesan cheese and bake in a preheated oven at 400° F for 30 minutes until golden brown.

Happiness's served!

Meatloaf

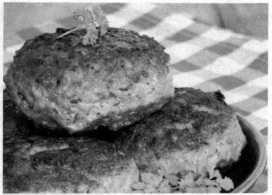

Ingredients for 4 portions:
- 3 cups minced beef
- 12 cups frozen spinach
- 2 cups zucchini
- 1 white egg
- 2 garlic cloves
- 1 spring parsley
- ¼ cup Evo oil
- Salt and pepper to taste

Nutrition 100 g:
Calories: 208 kcal **Carbs:** 2 g **Proteins:** 20 g **Fat:** 12 g
Directions:
1. Pour the minced meat and chopped parsley into a bowl.
2. Grate the zucchini and garlic inside. Add salt, pepper, egg white and ¼ cup oil. Mix everything with a ladle, then knead with your hands. Scald the spinach in the pot until cooked.
3. Then divide meat and spinach into 4 equal parts. Take one part of the meat and divide it further in half. Take one of the two halves and crush it on the palm of your hand and place the well-squeezed spinach in the center. Cover with the other part of the meat and form the first meatloaf.
4. Continue in this way in order to form 4 patties, placing them as you go on a baking sheet lined with parchment paper. Brush with the remaining oil and bake in a ventilated oven preheated to 360° F for 25 minutes. Remove from the oven and moisten the surface with the remaining sauce.
Meatloaf is like revenge, it's better when served… hot!

Cabbage and Lemon Salad

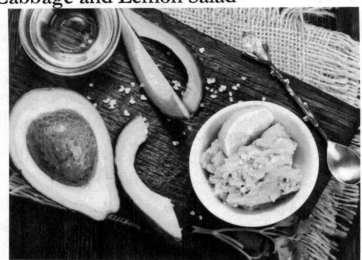

Ingredients for 4 portions:
- ½ cup water
- 1 garlic clove
- 1 tbsp lemon juice
- ½ tbsp fresh basil leaves
- 2 Avocados
- 400 g Cabbage salad
- ½ Evo oil
- 1 pinch salt
- Pepper to taste

Nutrition 100 g:
Calories: 179 kcal
Carbs: 5 g
Proteins: 8 g
Fat: 15 g
Directions:
1. Place basil and garlic in a mixer with a little bit of water, add the 2 avocados and lemon juice, mix until you get a cream.
2. In a bowl, prepare the cabbage salad and season with oil.
3. Season with the mixture you got and whisk well.
Too good to be true!

Greek Vegetables

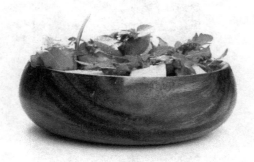

Ingredients for 2 portions:
- 2 tbsp of chia seeds
- 2 tbsp sesame seeds
- ½ onion, chopped
- 1 tsp garlic powder
- 1 cup feta cheese, sliced
- 1 red bell pepper, sliced
- ½ cup sliced mushrooms
- 1 bunch arugula
- 2 tbsp olive oil

Nutrition 100 g:
Calories: 235 kcal
Carbs: 5 g **Proteins:** 16 g
Fat: 18 g
Directions:
1.Combine seeds with the onion and garlic powder in a small bowl and dip the cheese slices into the bowl, then set aside in the refrigerator.
2. Place bell pepper and mushrooms in a skillet with oil over medium heat, without stirring, until they begin to brown and soften.
3. Meanwhile, place arugula on a plate. Add bell pepper and mushrooms on top of it.
4. Take the cheese from the refrigerator and lightly brown it for 30 seconds until it begins to melt.
5. Add the cheese slices to the salad and drizzle with olive oil.
You'll be dreaming of being in Greece!

Sandwich Bread

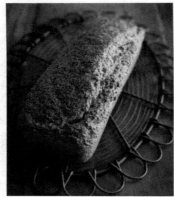

Ingredients (circa 20 slices):
- ¼ cup coconut flour
- 1 cup almond flour
- ½ flaxseed flour
- 1 tsp psyllium
- ½ cup clarified butter
- 3 eggs
- 1 cup lukewarm water
- 1 pinch dry yeast for bread
- 1 pinch seed – to decorate -
- Salt to taste - 3 g erythritol

Nutrition 100 g:
Calories: 341 kcal **Fat:** 18 g **Proteins:** 12 g **Carbs:** 5 g
Directions:
1. Preheat your oven at 400° F.
Combine all dry ingredients in a large bowl: flour, psyllium, baking powder, salt and erythritol.
3. Add eggs, butter and water and mix lightly with your hands.
4. Take a plum cake mold or baking sheet with baking paper and pour the dough.
5. Sprinkle with the seed mix and bake for about 25'.
6. Wait for it to cool a bit, then remove it from the mold.
7. If you want to, cut it into slices and put them back in the oven for another 5' in order to dry any moisture.
Best bread in the world!

Keto Pizza

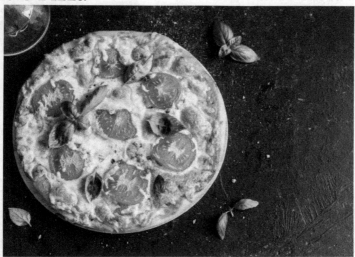

Ingredients 1 pizza:

- 4 cup cabbage or zucchini
- 1 egg
- ½ cup tomato sauce
- 1 mozzarella or braid
- Oregano, oil, salt to taste

Nutrition 100 g:

Calories: 351 kcal

Fat: 12 g

Proteins: 28 g

Carbs: 5 g

Directions:

1. Boil the cabbage or zucchini and let cool well.
2. Once cool, blend and squeeze into a cotton dishtowel.
3. Combine the blended vegetable with an egg.
4. Preheat your oven at 400° F, possibly ventilated.
5. Spread the dough on baking paper and cook for 20 minutes.
6. Add some sauce, mozzarella (cubed), oregano, oil. Add, if desired, a few slices of lean or cooked ham.
7. Bake in a ventilated oven for 10 minutes at 400° F.

Pizzaaaaaaaa!

Zucchini Lasagna

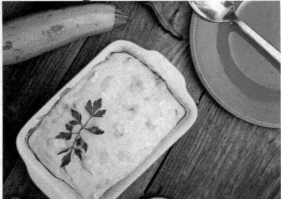

Ingredients for 2 portions:
- 4 and ¼ cups zucchini
- 1 egg
- ¼ grated cheese (Grana)
- 1 mozzarella
- 1 tbsp Evo oil
- Salt and pepper to taste

Nutrition for portion:
Calories: 440 kcal
Fat: 36 g
Proteins: 26 g
Carbs: 4 g
Directions:
1. Take the zucchini, wash them thoroughly, cut off the ends and rub them well on the cut side to reduce the bitter taste.
2. Grate the zucchini with a food grater.
3. In a bowl, combine the julienned zucchini with the egg and pour in the grated grana cheese, a pinch of salt and pepper, mix well.
4. Preheat the oven to 360° F.
5. Oil the bowl with a tablespoon of olive oil, pour the mixture evenly into the bowl using a spatula.
5. Bake and cook for 25 minutes at 360° F.
6. Meanwhile, cut the mozzarella into thin slices.
7. After 15 minutes, take out the terrine and arrange the mozzarella, bake, and finish cooking.
Enjoy a new type of drug!

Imperial Flatbread

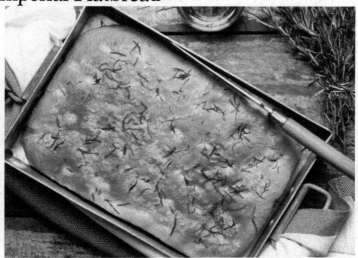

Ingredients for 2 portions:

- 1 cup almond flour
- 1 cup egg whites
- ¼ cup parmesan (better if there's no lactose)
- 2 tbsp Evo oil
- Salt, rosemary and pepper to taste

Nutrition 1 flatbread:

Calories: 650 kcal

Carbs: 4 g

Fat: 51 g

Proteins: 32 g

Directions:

1. Help yourself with a whisk and beat the egg whites and add almond flour, parmesan cheese. Mix well with a fork.

2. Lay it on baking paper, complete with oil, rosemary, salt.

3. Put it in the oven and cook for 15-20 minutes at 400° F.

Doesn't it sound like a dream?!

Shrimps with Sauce and Merengue

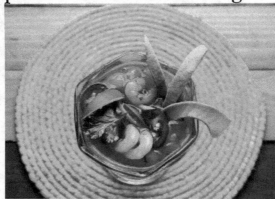

Ingredients 1 portion:

- 10 raw or cooked shrimps
- 1 avocado
- 1 tomato
- 1 tsp lemon juice
- 1 green chili pepper
- 10 gr shallot or spring onion
- Salt and pepper to taste
- 1 tbsp Evo oil
- 1 tsp valerian to garnish (optional)

Nutrition 100 g:

Calories: 271 kcal **Fat:** 26 g **Proteins:** 31 g
Carbs: 2 g

Directions:

1. Peel the avocado and remove its bone. Sprinkle avocado flesh with lemon juice. Add salt and pepper.
2. Chop shallot and add it to the avocado pulp, mashing it with a fork, together with the diced tomato and the previously emptied and diced chili.
3. Add 1 tbsp of Evo oil.
4. If you'd like a more creamy and homogeneous consistency, you can blend everything in a mixer.
5. Place the sauce in the middle of a plate, add shrimps and serve with a salad.

A delight for your palate!

Parmesan Eggplant

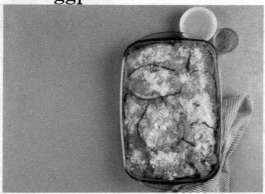

Ingredients for 4-5 Portions:
- 2 Eggplants
- 2 and ½ cup sausage
- 1 cup and ½ provola or Emmenthal cheese
- 2 cups cherry tomatoes
- 2 garlic gloves
- ½ cup Grana cheese
- 1 bunch rocket salad
- 6 tbsp Evo oil
- Oregano, pepper, hot pepper, and salt to taste

Nutrition 100 g:
Calories: 421 kcal **Fat:** 36 g **Proteins:** 21 g **Carbs:** 3 g
Directions:
1. Wash and thinly slice the eggplants with salt, pepper, and a weight on top so that they lose all their water (at least 2 hours).
2. Fry the eggplant in a pan with plenty of oil, then drain on paper towels. In a pan with a little oil, fry the garlic and the chili pepper, after a few minutes, pour the tomato puree and season it with salt, pepper, oregano, chopped rocket, add the sausage and simmer for at least 40 minutes.
3 In a rectangular baking dish, spread a little tomato sauce on the bottom, then place a slice of eggplant, a slice of provola, some sausage sauce and parmesan cheese on top. Continue making this multilayer until all the ingredients are used up.
5. Bake the eggplant at 360° F for about 40 minutes with a generous sprinkling of Parmesan cheese. Pleasure is served!

Ham Chicken

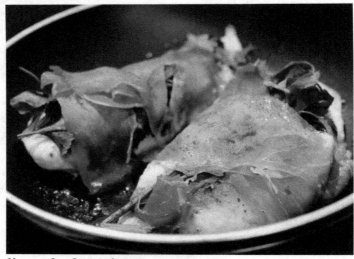

Ingredients for 2 portions:
- 2 chicken breasts
- 1 tbsp almonds
- 1 cup raw ham
- ½ cup Evo oil
- Bay leaf, salt and pepper to taste

Nutrition 100 g:
Calories: 281 kcal
Fat: 26 g
Proteins: 31 g
Carbs: 3 g

Directions:
1. Chop almonds with salt, pepper, and bay leaves in a blender.
2. Bread chicken breasts with the ingredients you just chopped, then place a slice of ham on every chicken breast and stop with a toothpick.
3. Cook for some minutes in a pan with hot oil or put them in the oven.
That will be a shock for your palate!

Mushrooms and Parmesan Salad

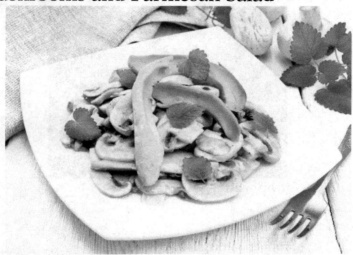

Ingredients for 1 portion:
- 1 cup fresh mushrooms
- 1/2 Avocado
- ¼ cup Parmesan, sliced
- 1 tsp Evo oil
- 1 tbsp lemon juice
- Parsley and salt to taste

Nutrition 100 g:
Calories: 271 kcal
Fat: 18 g
Proteins: 20 g
Carbs: 3 g
Directions:
1. Cut the mushrooms and the avocado into thin slices.
2. Combine oil, lemon, salt, and parsley.
3. Season mushrooms and avocado with the sauce, then add thin slices of parmesan.
A fresh and good meal!

The Baron's Cod

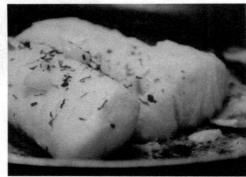

Ingredients for 1 portion:
- 1 cup cod
- 1 tbsp clarified butter
- 2 tsp chopped garlic cloves
- ½ tbsp mustard
- 1 shallot
- 1 tbsp Evo oil
- ½ tbsp lemon juice
- 1 tsp parsley
- Salt and pepper to taste

Nutrition 100 g:
Calories: 151 kcal
Fat: 8 g
Proteins: 22 g
Carbs: 2 g

Directions:
1. In a bowl, create a sauce by mixing butter, parsley, garlic, shallots, mustard, and lemon juice.
2. Heat the olive oil in a non-stick skillet over medium-high heat. Add the cod fillet.
3. Season fish with salt and pepper to taste.
4. Cook fillets for 3 to 4 minutes per side.
5. Preheat the oven to 440° F. Line a baking sheet with paper and place the fillets on it.
6. Arrange the prepared sauce evenly over the fillet.
7. Transfer to oven and bake for 5 to 10 minutes, or until fish is cooked through. Aristocrats are crazy about it!

Beef Medallions with Asparagus

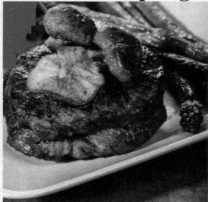

Ingredients for 1 portion:
- ½ cup medallions of beef
- ¼ cup chopped mushrooms
- ½ handful asparagus
- 2 tbsp coconut oil
- 1 tbsp chopped onion
- 1 tsp ginger
- 1 tsp parsley
- 2 cherry tomatoes, halved
- Salt and pepper to taste

Nutrition 100 g:
Calories: 178 kcal **Fat:** 10 g **Proteins:** 27 g
Carbs: 3 g

Directions:
1. Sprinkle the steaks with salt and pepper.
2. Heat some coconut oil in a skillet over medium heat, 2 minutes per side for a medium-cooked level. Cook longer if you prefer them well-done.
3. Remove the meat from the skillet. Grease with coconut oil and add onions.
4. Add asparagus, mushrooms and mix well in the same pan. Add the cherry tomatoes, parsley, and ginger. Stir well and cook until vegetables are tender.
5. Place the meat and veggies on a plate!
You'll be overwhelmed!

Parmesan Pizzas

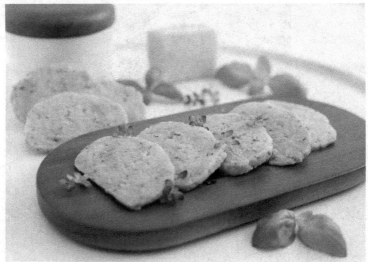

Ingredients for 1 portion:
- ½ cup grated Parmesan
- 2 tsp garlic cloves
- 2 tsp ground chili pepper
- 1 tsp chopped basil
- 1 tsp oregano
- Salt and pepper to taste

Nutrition 100 g:
Calories: 431 kcal
Fat: 29 g
Proteins: 38 g
Carbs: 1 g
Directions:
1. Preheat your oven at 360°. Place some baking sheet in a pan.
2. Place parmesan on the pan, shaping circles as thin as pancakes.
3. Season with species.
4. Bake for 5-7 minutes until they're brown.
5. You can also use them as snacks.
Best snack you've ever tried!

American Pizza

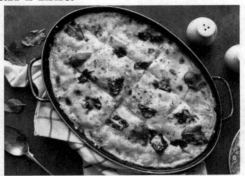

Ingredients for 1 portion:

- ½ cup minced meat
- 1/3 cup mushrooms
- 3 tbsp cubed mozzarella cheese
- 2 cups spinach
- 1 and ½ cup clarified butter
- 1 tsp oregano
- 1 tsp chopped garlic
- 1 spring basil
- Salt and pepper to taste

Nutrition 100 g:

Calories: 228 kcal **Fat:** 16 g **Proteins:** 26 g **Carbs:** 2 g

Directions:

1. Combine meat, oregano, basil, salt, and pepper in a bowl and mix well.
2. Preheat your oven at 400° F.
3. Press the mixture well with your hands in order to form a nice, rounded shape. Place the "pizza-meat" on a baking sheet lined with baking paper.
4. Bake in the preheated oven for 10-15 minutes.
5. In the meantime, grease a skillet with butter and heat it over high heat. Add garlic and mushrooms and cook for 5 minutes, often mixing. Add spinach and cook for an additional minute. Add salt and pepper. Set aside. Place half mozzarella on top of the meat. Add mushrooms and spinach. Add the other half of mozzarella on top.
6. Cook for 5 more minutes until the mozzarella melts. This is how a real American eats his pizza!

Mini Zucchini Hamburger

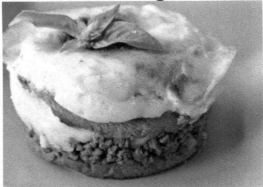

Ingredients for 1 portion:
- ½ cup minced meat
- 1 cup zucchini cut into thick slices
- 2 tbsp Evo oil
- 1 tbsp mayo (better if homemade)
- Salt, pepper, and mustard to taste

Nutrition 100 g:
Calories: 248 kcal
Fat: 20 g
Proteins: 24 g
Carbs: 3 g

Directions:
1. Preheat your oven at 400° F.
2. Grease a skillet with olive oil and sprinkle salt and pepper.
3. Place there the slices of zucchini.
4. Shape some meatballs, flatten them and put them in the skillet.
5. Place the skillet in the oven and cook for 15 minutes.
6. Put the meat between 2 slices of zucchini and add mayo and mustard.
7. Cook for some more minutes until the hamburgers become brown.
8. You can also double layer!
9. Stop with a toothpick.
It's going to be your challenge to McDonald's!

Fried Seabass

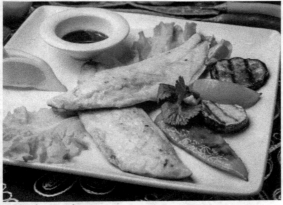

Ingredients for 1 portion:
- 1 cup seabass fillet (or sea bream)
- 2 tbsp clarified butter
- 2 tsp chopped garlic
- Salt and pepper to taste

Nutrition 100 g:
Calories: 218 kcal
Fat: 18 g
Proteins: 27 g
Carbs: 1 g
Directions:
1. Melt the butter in a frying pan.
2. Arrange fillets in a skillet and cook over medium-high heat.
3. Add minced garlic.
4. Sprinkle with salt, pepper, and garlic. As the fish cooks, it will go from being translucent to a solid white color. Wait for the white color to show through until halfway through the fillet, then flip it over and add the rest of the garlic.
5. Cook until the entire fillet turns a solid white color (it should flake easily).
6. Serve with a little garlic and butter from the pan.
Kids are crazy about it!

English Beef

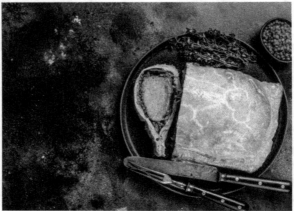

Ingredients for 1 portion:
- ½ cup steak fillet, halved
- 2 tbsp mozzarella, minced
- 2 tbsp almond flour
- 1 tbsp clarified butter
- 1 tbsp liver pate
- Salt and pepper to taste

Nutrition 100 g:
Calories: 298 kcal **Fat:** 16 g **Proteins:** 30 g **Carbs:** 3 g
Directions:
1. Marinade meat with salt and pepper.
2. Melt butter over medium-high heat and add the marinated beef.
3. Let the steaks cool and at the same time heat the mozzarella cheese in the microwave for about 1 minute.
4. Mix the mozzarella cheese with the almond flour until it forms a paste.
5. Place the dough on a piece of parchment paper, use another piece of parchment paper over the dough and a rolling pin to flatten it. Remove the second piece of baking paper and spread some butter over the dough.
6. Place the meat in one end of the dough and roll up the dough and meat. Preheat the oven to 400° F. Line a baking sheet with baking paper and place the dough on it.
8. Bake for about 25-30 minutes or until the "dough" is golden brown. You have no idea what you're going to eat!

Delivery Pizza

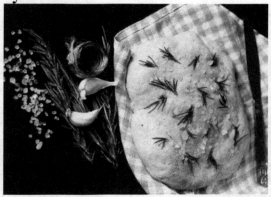

Ingredients:
- 1 egg
- ½ cup egg white
- ½ cup yogurt
- Salt, rosemary and species

Nutrition 100 g:
Calories: 293 kcal **Fat:** 12 g **Proteins:** 32 g
Carbs: 5 g
Directions:
1. Preheat your oven at 360° F.
2. Combine the egg yolk with the yogurt and spices in a bowl.
3. In a different bowl, whip the egg whites until stiff (they're ready when, removing the whisk, the so-called pico de gallo remains on them).
4. Incorporate the yogurt and yolk mixture into the whipped egg whites, from the bottom upwards, preferably by hand or with a silicone paddle, gently so as not to disassemble the mixture. The purpose of this operation is to incorporate air.
5. Line a baking sheet with parchment paper, and place the mixture in a round shape, about two fingers thick as desired.
6. Bake, baking for 15 minutes.
7. Remove from oven, add a drizzle of oil and rosemary, or season to taste, such as sliced tomato and anchovies, or tomato and mozzarella.
We're Neapolitans, folks!

Sesame Buns for Hamburgers

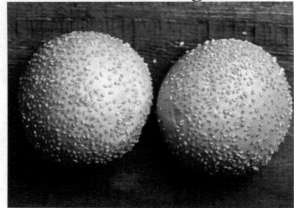

Ingredients:
- 2 egg yolks
- 2 egg whites
- 2 tbsp cream cheese
- 1 tbsp toasted sesame seeds
- ½ tsp baking powder
- 1 tbsp olive oil

Nutrition 100 g:
Calories: 189 kcal
Fat: 12 g
Proteins: 22 g
Carbs: 2 g
Directions:
1. Beat egg whites and baking powder until egg whites are whipped.
2. Heat cream cheese in your microwave on medium-low intensity for about 30 seconds, 10 seconds at a time, until softened. Stir with a spoon and set aside to let cool.
3. Mix the egg yolks with the melted cream cheese.
4. Add beaten eggs and cheese mixture to egg whites. Combine compounds, stirring gently.
5. Preheat your oven at 380° F. Cover the baking sheet with baking paper and brush it with oil. Add the dough.
6. Shape balls, no matter the size. Sprinkle with sesame seeds.
7. Bake for about 18-20 minutes or until golden brown.
Now you can make yourself any type of sandwich!

Keto Bread

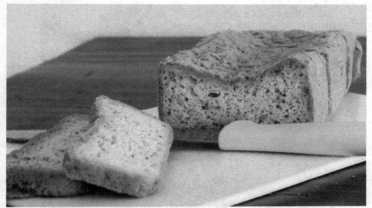

Ingredients for 1 portion:

- ¼ cup almond flour
- 1 tsp psyllium powder
- 1 tsp baking powder
- Salt to taste
- ¼ cup water
- ½ egg white

Nutrition 100 g:
Calories: 424 kcal
Fat: 36 g
Proteins: 22 g
Carbs: 5 g
Directions:
1. Preheat the oven at 380° F.
2. Combine the dry ingredients in a big bowl, remembering that these are for 1 sandwich only, increasing the amount in portion to how many you want to make.
3. Add boiled water and white eggs to a bowl. In the meantime, beat eggs with a mixer for about 30 seconds until the dough begins to have consistency.
4. Moisten your hands and shake the dough.
5. Arrange on a greased baking sheet. Bake on a lower rack for 50-60 minutes. They're done when you hear a hollow sound when you touch the bottom of the loaf.
Eating bread and butter without getting fat: a dream come true!

Chicken Fries

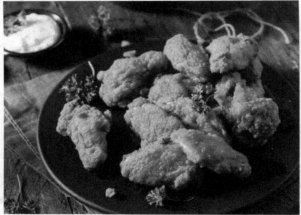

Ingredients for 2 portions:
- 2 chicken breasts
- ½ red onion
- Parsley, rosemary (fresh or dried)
- 1 beaten egg
- Almond flour to bread
- Juice of ½ lemon
- Nutmeg, pepper and salt to taste

Nutrition 100 g:
Calories: 424 kcal
Fat: 36 g
Proteins: 22 g
Carbs: 5 g

Directions:
1. Mince chicken. Chop the onion, rosemary and parsley and set them aside, you'll need them later.
2. Combine chicken and onion, rosemary, salt, and pepper in a bowl. Add the beaten egg to the nutmeg and then whisk well.
3. Bread the morsels in the almond flour, shaping them as you wish.
4. Fry or bake until golden brown. Let cool and then make portions and sprinkle the chopped ingredients left aside over the morsels and serve.

A delight for your eyes, nose, and mouth!

Vegetable Fries

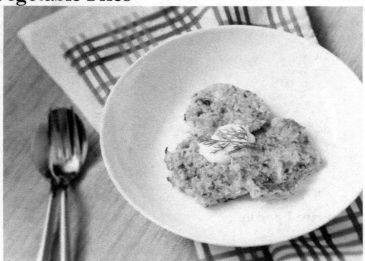

Ingredients for 1 portion:
- 2 eggs
- 1 tbsp coconut flour
- ½ tsp instant yeast (optional)
- Cooked vegetables to taste (choose between herbs, spinach, carrots, zucchini, peppers)
- 1 tbsp olive oil
- Salt and pepper to taste

Nutrition 100 g:
Calories: 274 kcal
Fat: 18 g
Proteins: 16 g
Carbs: 4 g
Directions:
1. Whisk two eggs with a tablespoon of coconut flour and a bunch of powder.
2. Add steamed, drained, and salted vegetables. Cut it and then cook as if they were pancakes, wetting the pan with oil – if necessary.
3. Cook until golden brown.
Here's your engine!

Russian Salad with Salmon

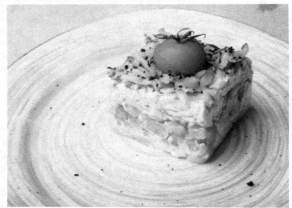

Ingredients for 1 portion:

- ½ cup salmon
- ¼ cup carrots
- 20 gr cooked red turnips
- 25 g Avocado
- Mayo without sugar, 20 gr
- Hemp seeds
- ¼ cup olive oil
- Salt and pepper to taste

Nutrition:

Calories: 434 kcal

Fat: 40,9 g

Carbs: 4,2 g

Proteins: 12,3 g

Directions:

1. Cut turnips, carrots, and the avocado into cubes, combine mayonnaise and oil, adjust salt and pepper, and your coleslaw is ready.

2. Cook the salmon in a non-stick pan, turning it over a couple of times until it's crispy on both sides; use a silicone spatula to avoid leaving any grease on the pan.

3. Now, if you want, you can either cut the salmon into small cubes and put it in a salad or eat them separately.

Doesn't it feel like eating with the Tsar?

The Pirate's Swordfish

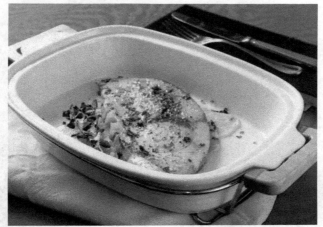

Ingredients for 2 portions:

- 2 fresh swordfish fillets (about 300 g)
- 2 tbsp olive oil
- 1 spring fresh marjoram
- 1 spring fresh mint
- 1 tsp coriander seeds
- 1 tsp ginger powder
- 1 tbsp lemon peel
- Salt and pepper to taste

Nutrition 1 portion:
Calories: 385 kcal
Carbs: 1 g
Fat: 30 g
Proteins: 28 g
Directions:
1. Grind the coriander seeds in a mortar with the ginger powder, then place the salmon fillets on a baking sheet lined with baking paper and sprinkle with the freshly made spice powder, marjoram, chopped mint and grated lemon peel.
2. Season with salt and a drizzle of oil.
3. Bake at 360° F for 15 minutes.
4. Add raw olive oil if you want to.
Let's get ready... time to eat!

Mediterranea Hake

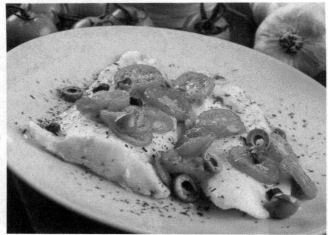

Ingredients for 4 portions:
- 6 cups fresh hake, already cleaned (hake or cod)
- 4 tbsp olive oil
- 1 tbsp black olives
- 1 tbsp desalted capers
- ½ cup cherry tomatoes
- 1 pinch fresh parsley
- Salt and pepper to taste

Nutrition for each portion
Calories: 236 kcal
Carbs: 1 g
Fat: 16 g
Proteins: 34 g
Directions:
1. Clean the hake by removing the heads, guts and central bone or have them cleaned at the fishmonger.
2. Prepare a baking tray and line some baking paper on it. Place the fish open in half with the body facing one another.
3. Add halved cherry tomatoes, capers, whole black olives, and sprinkle chopped parsley. Drizzle with oil and salt.
4. Cook for 20 minutes at 400° F.
You'll taste the best sea flavors!

Lemon Bream

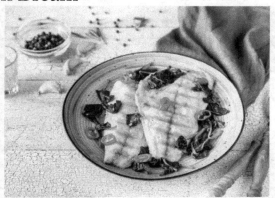

Ingredients for 2 portions:

- 2 giltheads, already cleaned, or 4 fillets (you can also use sea bass)
- 2 lemons
- 1 spring parsley
- 1 tbsp coriander seeds
- 2 tbsp extra virgin olive oil
- Salt and pepper to taste

Nutrition for 1 portion:
Calories: 294 kcal **Carbs:** 4 g **Fat:** 12 g **Proteins:** 38 g

Directions:

1. Wash the already cleaned gilthead seabreams and lay them on a baking sheet covered with baking paper.

2. Slice 1 lemon into thin slices and place them inside the bream together with a sprig of parsley.

3. Bake the sea bream at 400° F for 20 minutes.

4. In the meantime, prepare the dressing: squeeze the remaining lemon and place the juice in a small bowl. Add a pinch of salt and pepper and whisk with a fork, adding the extra virgin olive oil. Chop the coriander seeds and add them to the emulsion along with some finely chopped parsley. When the fish is cooked, clean it by removing the skin to obtain fillets on which you will pour the lemon and coriander. If you wish, you can add more fresh parsley.

6. Serve with a side dish of cooked seasonal vegetables (artichokes, green beans, grilled zucchini) or a mixed salad.

Taste one of the best Mediterranean fish!

Creamy Chicken with Garlic

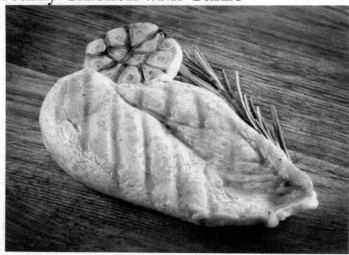

Ingredients for 1 portion:

- 1 chicken breast (big)
- ¼ cup butter
- 1 garlic clove
- 1 tbsp extra virgin olive oil
- Salt and pepper to taste

Nutrition 100 g:
Calories: 491 kcal
Fat: 31 g
Proteins: 52 g
Carbs: 1 g
Directions:
1. Peel and mince the garlic clove.
2. In a small saucepan, melt the butter over low heat.
3. Combine melted butter, garlic clove, salt and pepper and set aside this creamy mixture you've created.
4. In a skillet, heat the oil and fry the chicken breast until cooked on each side.
5. Place the chicken breast on a dish and sprinkle it with the mixture of butter and garlic.
Enjoy!

Salmon on Cabbage

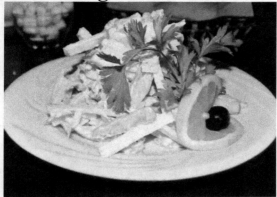

Ingredients for 1 portion:
- 1 fillet salmon
- 1 cup cabbage
- 1 and ½ tbsp butter
- 1 pinch coconut cream, without sugars
- 2 tbsp extra virgin olive oil
- Turmeric to taste
- Garlic powder to taste

Nutrition 100 g:
Calories: 451 kcal
Fat: 59 g
Proteins: 32 g
Carbs: 3 g
Directions:
1. Cut salmon into small pieces and drizzle with 1 tablespoon oil.
2. In a bowl, mix the coconut cream with turmeric and garlic powder.
3. Dip the salmon into the coconut cream.
4. In a skillet, cook the salmon until golden brown, after which cover with foil and set aside.
5. Melt the butter in a skillet, fry the cabbage until it begins to brown slightly and place it on a plate.
6. Lay the salmon on the cabbage bed and drizzle with the rest of the extra virgin olive oil.
Out of this world!

King's Pork Chop

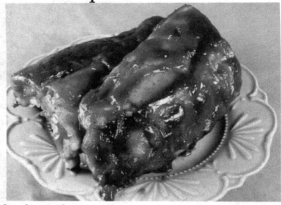

Ingredients for 1 portion:
- 2 cups pork chop
- 2 tbsp mustard
- 1 tsp ghee butter
- 2 garlic cloves
- Paprika, pepper, salt, rosemary, and chili pepper to taste

Nutrition 100 g:
Calories: 499 kcal
Fat: 40 g
Proteins: 53 g
Carbs: 2 g
Directions:
1. Rub the chops with a garlic clove.
2. Preheat your oven at 400° F.
3. Put the mustard in a bowl.
4. Mince the second garlic clove with a knife.
5. Combine paprika, garlic clove, pepper, salt, and chili pepper in another bowl.
6. Place a sheet of foil next to both bowls.
7. Dip 1 chop in the mustard and species mixture and place on the foil.
8. Add butter on top.
9. Wrap it in the foil and put it on a baking sheet.
10. Cook for 60 minutes.
Mouthwatering!

Tuna Fillet in Green Fields

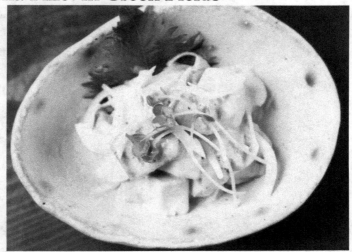

Ingredients for 1 portion:
- 1 cup fillet tuna
- 1 tbsp mayo
- 1/2 avocado, sliced
- 1 cup salad
- 1 tbsp Evo oil
- 1/2 onion
- Salt and pepper to taste

Nutrition 100 g:
Calories: 285 kcal
Fat: 29 g
Proteins: 26 g
Carbs: 3 g
Directions:
1. Season the chopped onion in a bowl with oil, pepper, and salt.
2. Cut the tuna and the avocado into slices (as you wish).
3. Place the seasoned salad in a dish next to the avocado.
4. Place the tuna on ton and season with mayo.
Enjoy a very smart meal!

Speck and Salmon Skewer

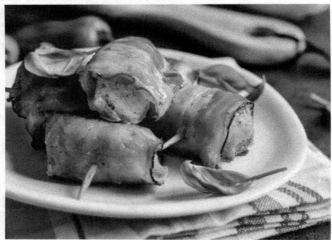

Ingredients for 4 portions:

- 1 cup speck
- 1 tsp minced basil
- pepper
- 3 cup salmon
- 1 tbsp Evo oil
- 8 wooden sticks

Nutrition 100 g:

Calories: 284 kcal

Fat: 29 g

Proteins: 26 g

Carbs: 0 g

Directions:

1. Take the wooden skewers and wet them under running water.

2. Take the basil leaves and chop them finely.

3. Cut the salmon into strips.

4. Dip the salmon in basil and add pepper if you like.

5. Cut speck into strips.

6. Roll salmon around the skewers and add speck on top of the salmon.

7. Pour extra virgin olive oil on them.

8. Cook in the oven or in a pan, as you prefer.

Dish's served!

Cheesy Meatballs

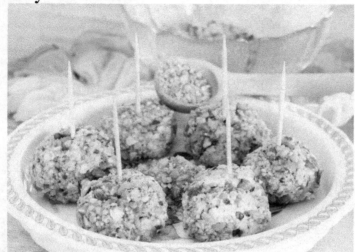

Ingredients for 4 portions:
- ½ cup goat cheese
- 1 tbsp pistachio
- 1 tbsp almonds
- Salt and pepper to taste

Nutrition 100 g:
Calories: 340 kcal
Fat: 30 g
Proteins: 22 g
Carbs: 1 g
Directions:
1. Divide the goat cheese and shape balls.
2. Mince almonds and pistachios.
3. Add salt and pepper.
4. Pour this powder into a bowl and roll the cheese pieces on them so that they will flavor and become delicious.
It's raining meatballs!

Sausage and Onion Pie

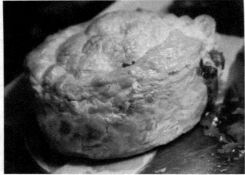

Ingredients for 4 portions:
- 1 cup almond flour
- 1 cup pork sausage - 1 onion
- ½ cup milk without sugar
- 1 egg - 1 tsp garlic powder
- Salt and pepper to taste - 1 tbsp Evo oil
- 1 tbsp fresh spinach
- 2 tbsp cheese, grated

Nutrition 100 g:
Calories: 567 kcal **Fat:** 30 g **Proteins:** 29 g **Carbs:** 5 g
Directions:
1. Preheat the oven at 360° F.
2. Pour a drizzle of oil into a frying pan and brown the onion (that you've already cut into squares) with the sausage paste.
3. Pour the almond flour into a bowl with a tablespoon of garlic powder and almond milk. Mix well until everything is combined.
4. Add grated cheese and egg and continue to mix until you get a dough.
5. Take a baking pan of about 8 inches and cover it with baking paper, pour the dough on top and spread it out by pressing it with your fingers evenly. It must maintain a thickness of about 0,60 inches. Place fresh spinach, salt, pepper, sausage paste with onion and extra virgin olive oil on top of the dough. Fold the edge of the savory pie dough over the filling, creating the shape of a real pie.
7. Using a brush, brush the pie with olive oil. Bake for 25-30 minutes, it's ready when the dough turns golden brown.
Finger-licking good!

Spinach Omelet

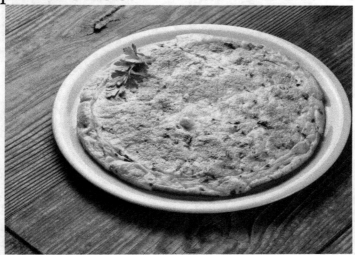

Ingredients for 1 portion:

- 2 eggs
- 1 tbsp coconut or Evo oil
- ½ tbsp turmeric
- ½ cup spinach
- Salt and pepper to taste

Nutrition 100 g:
Calories: 278 kcal
Carbs: 3 g
Proteins: 20 g
Fat: 18 g
Directions:
1. Add the eggs, spinach, turmeric, pepper and salt in a blender and mix.
2. Heat the oil in a skillet over medium heat.
3. Pour the resulting egg-mixture and cook for 2-3 minutes. With the help of a lid, flip the omelet on the other side and cook for 2 minutes more.

If you want to make an omelet, you've got to break some eggs!

Tuna and Eggs Salad

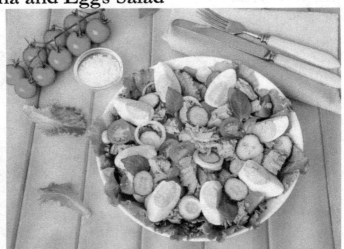

Ingredients for 4 portions:

- 1 and ½ cup tuna in oil (drained)
- 4 eggs
- 2 cucumbers
- 4 tomatoes
- ½ lettuce
- 1 lemon, sliced
- 4 tbsp extra virgin olive oil
- Salt to taste

Nutrition 100 g:
Calories: 178 kcal
Carbs: 2 g
Proteins: 20 g
Fat: 12 g

Directions:

1. Wash the vegetable with baking soda if possible.
2. Cut into thin slices and place them in a big bowl.
3. Boil the eggs from 4 to 8 minutes, as you wish. Slice them and place them on the vegetables.
4. Place the tuna on the vegetables as well.
5. Combine, adding oil gradually. Add also salt and sprinkle lemon. A classic!

Pizza

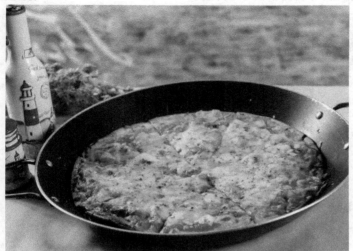

Ingredients for 1 portion:
- ½ cup egg whites
- 1 tbsp almond flour
- 1 tbsp coconut flour
- ½ cup tomato sauce
- ½ cup mozzarella (without milk)
- Salt, basil and your favorite spices (to taste)

Nutrition 100 g:
Calories: 180 kcal
Carbs: 5 g
Proteins: 23 g
Fat: 14 g

Directions:
1. Preheat a frying pan.
2. Combine all the ingredients in a bowl and mix well until you get a homogeneous mix.
3. Roll the mixture by hands or with a rolling pin to get a 0,20 inches thickness.
4. Pout in the pan and cook for a couple of minutes, then flip.
5. Season and cook for some more minutes (if you cover it with string cheese, cover the pan with a lid)
This is real Italy!

Light Russian Salad

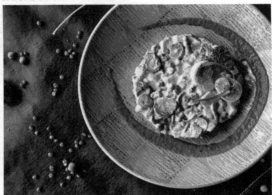

Ingredients for 1 portion:
- 1 raw potato with peel (120 gr)
- 1 raw potato with peel (120 gr)
- ½ cup cooked peas
- ½ cup pickled onions
- 2 tbsp. mayo without sugar
- ¼ cup Greek yogurt
- 2 eggs
- Salt and parsley to taste

Nutrition 100 g:
Calories: 125 kcal
Carbs: 7 g
Proteins: 24 g
Fat: 14 g

Directions:
1. Boil eggs for 5 minutes in hot water.
2. Slice one to decorate, cut the other one into little pieces.
3. Cook carrot and potato for 10-15 minutes, then cut them into cubes.
4. Add peas and chopped pickled onions.
5. Combine mayo and Greek yogurt in a bowl.
6. Add all the other ingredients and salt.
7. Serve in a dish and garnish with the first egg and parsley.
It's Beethoven's new symphony!

Queen's Cauliflower Soup

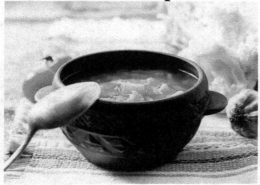

Ingredients for 3 portions:

- 2 onions, diced
- 5 tomatoes, diced
- 1 cauliflower head
- 1 tbsp pistachio
- 1 tsp chopped ginger
- 1 tsp chopped garlic
- 3 tbsp of Evo oil
- 1 bay leaf - ½ tsp cumin seeds
- ¼ tbsp pepper and salt to taste
- 1 green and 2 black cardamom
- 3 cloves - 1 tsp of turmeric
- 2 cups hot water

Nutrition 100 g:
Calories: 177 kcal **Carbs:** 4 g **Proteins:** 6 g **Fat:** 18 g
Directions:
1. Preheat a pot with oil. Add the cumin seeds, black cardamom, the bay leaf, green cardamom, pepper, and cloves.
2. Sauté for 30 seconds and add the onions, garlic, and ginger. Stir for 5 minutes and add the spices. Cook for 2 minutes and add tomatoes, stirring. Add pistachios.
3. Blend the mixture using a blender.
4. Put everything in a pot and slowly add hot water, stirring the mixture continuously. Add the cauliflower to the mixture and put the lid on the pot. Cook over medium heat for 10 minutes.
We're ready, aren't we?!

Dancing Zucchini

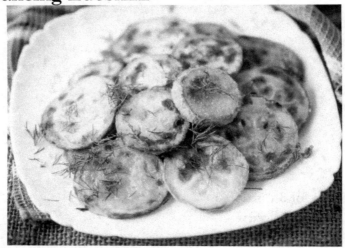

Ingredients for 2 portions:

- 2 zucchinis
- 4 tbsp Evo oil
- 2 minced garlic cloves
- 1 lemon zest
- 1 tbsp lemon juice
- Salt and pepper to taste

Nutrition 100 g:
Calories: 97 kcal
Carbs: 1 g
Proteins: 1 g
Fat: 9 g
Directions:
1. Heat the oil in a pan over medium-high heat and sauté the lemon zest and the minced garlic.
2. Cut the zucchini into thin slices and place them on the pan, adding salt and pepper to taste. Sprinkle lemon juice on it and cook for 2 minutes.

To eat in a heartbeat!

Bolshevik Shrimps

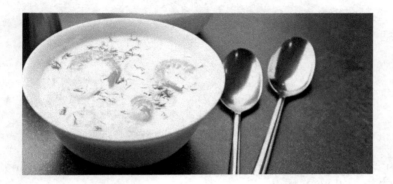

Ingredients for 1 portion:
- 1 cup shrimps, shelled
- 1 cup ricotta cheese or Greek yogurt
- 3 red radicchio leaves
- 3 tbsp cooking cream (sugar-free)
- Vinegar, salt and pepper to taste

Nutrition 100 g:
Calories: 393 kcal
Fat: 30 g
Proteins: 36 g
Carbs: 5 g
Directions:
1. Cook the shrimps (even frozen) and put them in a bowl. Add the chopped radicchio, a couple of drops of vinegar and mix everything.
2. Add the ricotta cheese and mix, add salt and pepper and mix until you get a homogeneous mixture. Keep it in the fridge until you're ready to use it.
A delicious cream!

Tuna Sauce

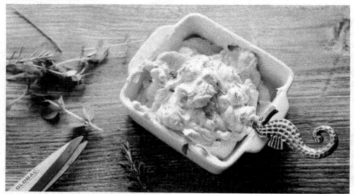

A special meal that can be used to serve meat or salad, using as much as you want of it.

Ingredients:

- 2 zucchinis (only pulp)
- 1 cup tuna with olive oil
- 2 anchovies
- Salt and pepper to taste
- 1 tsp mustard

Nutrition 100 g:
Calories: 147 kcal
Fat: 3 g
Proteins: 24 g
Carbs: 2 g

Directions:
1. Blend all the ingredients.
2. Keep it in the fridge.
You'll be on top of the world!

Southern Italy Spicy Chicken

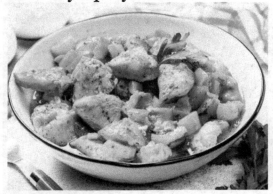

Ingredients for 1 portion:

- 1 cup of chicken, cubed
- 2 tbsp coconut oil
- 1 green pepper
- 1 tbsp crushed garlic
- 1 tbsp crushed red pepper
- 1 tbsp Evo oil
- 1 tbsp mustard
- Salt and pepper to taste
- ½ avocado
- 1 tbsp lemon juice (lime is better)

Nutrition 100 g:

Calories: 173 kcal

Fat: 10 g

Proteins: 21 g

Carbs: 2 g

Directions:

1. Cut chicken into little pieces and mix with garlic, pepper, oil, and mustard.

2. Fry the chicken in coconut oil over medium heat.

3. When the chicken's ready, place it on a plate and serve with raw bell pepper and diced avocado with salt, pepper, and lime juice.

Fire will come out of your mouth!

Squash Blossoms in Love

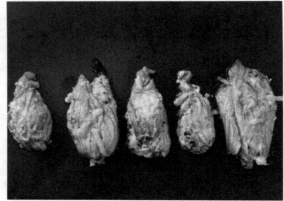

Ingredients for 2 portions:
- 10 squash blossoms
- 1 cup ricotta
- ½ cup grated parmesan
- 1 egg
- 1 tbsp Evo oil
- Salt and pepper to taste

Nutrition 100 g:
Calories: 253 kcal
Fat: 20 g
Proteins: 21 g
Carbs: 1 g
Directions:
1. Mix ricotta cheese, parmesan cheese and the egg in a bowl. Add salt, pepper (and any other spice, if desired).
2. Wash squash blossoms and gently pat dry with kitchen paper and remove their inner pistil, trying not to break them.
3. Prepare a piping bag with the cheese mixture, if not, use your fingers, stuff the flowers, and place them on a sheet of baking paper with which you have lined the baking dish.
4. If you want, you can brush them with some olive oil.
5. Put them in a static oven and cook for 15-20 minutes at 360° F.
So tasty!

Super Mayo

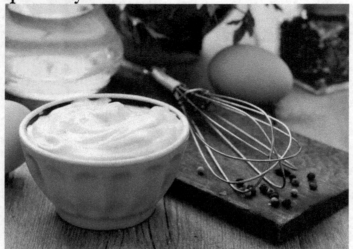

Ingredients:

- 1 cup Evo oil
- 1/3 cup almond milk without sugar
- 1 tbsp apple vinegar
- 1 tsp mustard
- 1 spring rosemary
- 4 basil leaves
- 3 sage leaves
- 10 drops of lemon
- Salt and pepper to taste

Nutrition 100 g:
Calories: 808 kcal
Fat: 80 g
Proteins: 5 g
Carbs: 1 g
Directions:
1. Wash, dry, mince the herbs in a blender, pouring milk, mustard, vinegar, and lemon drops. Add some oil and salt and pepper.
2. Blend until mayo is congealed. Serve cold.
Finger-licking!

Curry Chicken

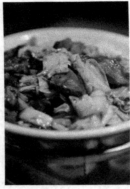

Ingredients for 1 portion:
- 2 tbsp coconut oil
- 1 cup chicken breast
- 1 red bell pepper, chopped
- ½ cucumber, diced
- 1 tsp pumpkin seeds
- 1 tbsp blueberries
- 30 g Salad (optional)
- 2 tbsp olive oil
- 1 tsp finely chopped coriander
- Salt, black pepper and curry powder to taste

Nutrition 100 g:
Calories: 198 kcal
Fat: 16 g
Proteins: 25 g
Carbs: 3 g
Directions:
1. Preheat a skillet over medium-high heat and cook the cubed chicken in coconut oil until golden brown.
2. Arrange the chicken pieces in a bowl and let them cool for a few minutes. Add diced bell pepper, cucumber or zucchini, pumpkin seeds, and blueberries to the bowl. Stir in the oil, curry powder, salt, pepper, and chopped cilantro.
3. Serve with salad leaves or on its own.
Curious meal!

Salmon Soup

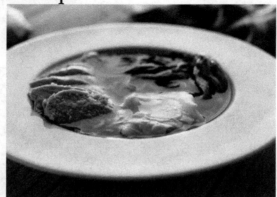

Ingredients for 2 portions:

- 2 eggs
- ½ cup zucchini
- 1 and 1/3 cup salmon
- 1 and ½ chicken stock
- 2 cups minced spinach
- ½ lemon juice
- 2 tsp garlic
- Salt and pepper to taste

Nutrition 100 g:
Calories: 197 kcal
Fat: 10 g
Proteins: 24 g
Carbs: 2 g
Directions:
1. Pour the chicken stock into a saucepan and begin to heat it.
2. Chop the zucchini and garlic and add them along with the broth.
3. Cut the salmon into strips or chunks and pour into the saucepan.
4. Add the lemon juice.
5. Add salt and pepper to taste.
6. Crack 2 eggs into the same saucepan and let them poach. Cook until liquid is almost completely evaporated.
A healthy meal!

Lemon Chicken

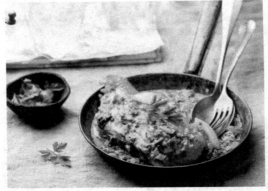

Ingredients for 1 portion:
- ½ cup of chicken stock
- 1 cup chicken breast or thighs
- 1 and ½ tbsp butter
- 1 tbsp Evo oil
- 1 tsp garlic
- 1 tsp basil
- 1 tsp oregano
- Salt and pepper to taste
- Juice of ½ lemon

Nutrition 100 g:
Calories: 227 kcal
Fat: 14 g
Proteins: 24 g
Carbs: 2 g
Directions:
1. Heat the olive oil in a skillet over medium-high heat.
2. Add chicken breasts and season on both sides with salt, pepper, oregano, and basil.
3. Cook for 2-3 minutes per side until browned.
4. Transfer chicken to a baking dish.
5. In a bowl, mix butter, garlic, chicken broth and lemon juice.
6. Pour the mixture over the chicken. Cook for 20-30 minutes until the chicken is cooked. Spoon the pan juices over the chicken on a plate, then sprinkle with parsley and serve. Garnish with lemon slices, if desired. It was also known as the Duke's dinner!

Delicious Brie

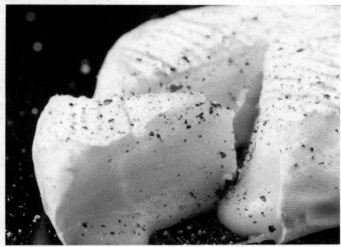

Ingredients for 1 portion:
- 1/3 cup of Brie cheese
- 1 tbsp olive oil
- Parsley and pepper to taste

Nutrition 100 g:
Calories: 417 kcal
Fat: 28 g
Proteins: 21 g
Carbs: 0 g
Directions:
1. Remove the rind from the cheese and dice it.
2. Place a few pieces of cheese on some baking paper on a plate and bake in the oven at medium temperature for 1-2 minutes, until melted.
3. Let them cool and sprinkle with oil and spices.
Easy, but mind-blowing!

Sea Meatballs

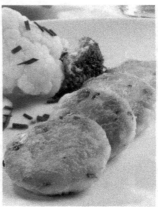

Ingredients for 1 portion:
- 1 egg yolk
- 1 cup cauliflower
- 1 cup salmon
- 1 tbsp clarified butter
- 30 gr cooking cream
- 2 tbsp olive oil
- Lemon juice, salt, and pepper to taste

Nutrition 100 g:
Calories: 417 kcal **Fat:** 28 g
Proteins: 21 g
Carbs: 0 g

Directions:

1. Cut the fish into small pieces and place them in a blender. Add egg yolks, cream, and spices.

2. Shape meatballs with wet hands.

3. Heat butter over medium heat until golden brown. Lower the heat and sauté the meatballs for a few more minutes until cooked through.

4. Roughly chop the cauliflower and place it in a large pot. Cover with water. Bring to a boil and add a generous pinch of salt. Lower the heat and simmer until the cauliflower is tender. Drain well.

5. Serve the salmon balls with the freshly boiled cauliflower, lemon or lime juice, pepper, and a drizzle of extra virgin olive oil.

One leads to another!

Devil's Chicken

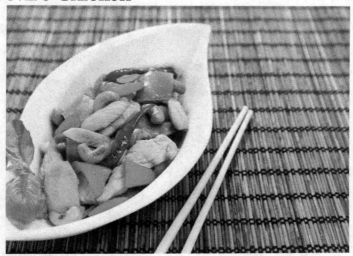

Ingredients for 1 portion:
- 1 cup chicken, cubed
- 2 tbsp cashews
- 2 tbsp soy sauce
- ½ medium cucumber, peeled and diced
- 2 tbsp coconut oil
- ½ tbsp vinegar
- 1 tsp chopped red chili pepper
- 2 tsp minced garlic (optional)

Nutrition 100 g:
Calories: 267 kcal
Fat: 18 g
Proteins: 24 g
Carbs: 2 g
Directions:
1. Sauté the diced chicken breast in coconut oil until cooked through. Remove from the heat and place on a plate.
2. Sauté the diced cucumber, cashews and chopped chili in coconut oil until softened a bit (5 minutes).
3. Add diced chicken, garlic, soy sauce and vinegar.
4. Sauté for another 5 minutes and serve.
You'll feel like a little devil after eating it!

Eskimo Salmon

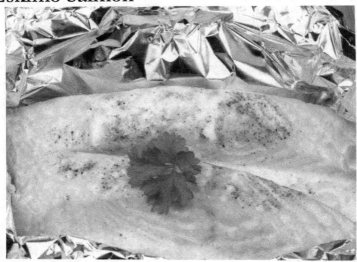

Ingredients for 1 portion:
- 1 cup fillet salmon
- 2 tbsp grated parmesan
- 2 tbsp clarified butter
- 2 tbsp mayo, better if homemade
- 2 tsp parsley
- 2 tsp minced garlic
- Salt and pepper to taste

Nutrition 100 g:
Calories: 274 kcal
Fat: 20 g
Proteins: 25 g
Carbs: 1 g
Directions:
1. Put the salmon in a pan lined with baking paper and season with salt and pepper.
2. Preheat the oven at 360° F.
3. Add butter and the remaining ingredients in a bowl and mix until they're very well amalgamated.
4. Pour this mixture on salmon.
5. Cook the salmon until you get to easily cut it with a fork.
Here you have some Alaskan flavors!

Chicken and Walnut Stews

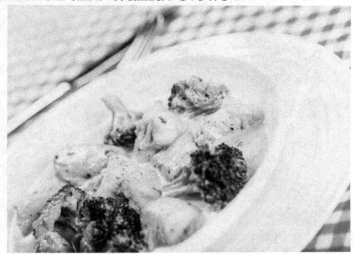

Ingredients for 1 portion:
- 1 cup chicken, diced
- 8 shelled walnuts
- 1/3 cup broccoli
- ¼ cup mayo, better if homemade
- 1 tbsp Evo oil
- Salt and pepper to taste

Nutrition 100 g:
Calories: 414 kcal
Fat: 36 g
Proteins: 25 g
Carbs: 3 g

Directions:
1. Heat a non-stick skillet over medium-high heat and lay the chicken nuggets in it.
2. Cook for 4-5 minutes or until golden brown.
3. Place broccoli in a small saucepan, add water and a pinch of salt. Boil for a few minutes until tender, evaporate water and toss with oil.
4. Add walnuts and cook until broccoli is crispy (but not boiled).
5. Serve the meat with broccoli and walnuts. Add mayonnaise and pepper, if desired.

You'll be seeing stars!

Tuna Hamburger

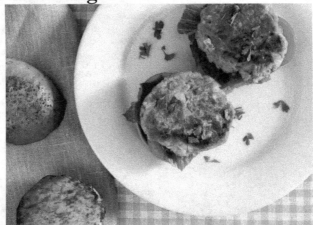

Ingredients for 1 portion:

- 2 tbsp coconut flour
- 1 cup tuna, fresh or canned
- 2 eggs
- 1 tbsp coconut oil
- 1 tbsp Evo oil
- 2 2 tbsp coconut flakes without sugar
- 1 tbsp fresh basil, finely chopped
- 1 tbsp chopped hot chili peppers
- salt

Nutrition 100 g:

Calories: 219 kcal

Fat: 18 g

Proteins: 28 g

Carbs: 2 g

Directions:

1. Cut the tuna into pieces.

2. Combine all the ingredients in a bowl.

3. Shape some hamburgers with the help of a scoop.

4. Add coconut oil into a skillet and cook over medium heat. Cook the hamburgers, flipping them on either side until golden brown. Serve hot either with keto bread or with vegetables.

What a Hamburger!

Avocado Cradle

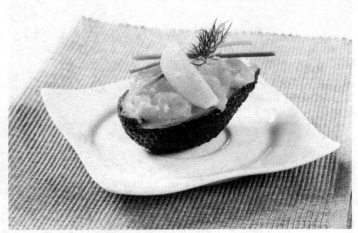

Ingredients for 1 portion:

- 1 cup smoked salmon
- ½ avocado
- 2 tbsp whipping cream without sugar
- Salt and pepper to taste

Nutrition 100 g:
Calories: 241 kcal
Fat: 10 g
Proteins: 26 g
Carbs: 3 g
Directions:
1. Cut the avocado in half and remove the seed.
2. Add cream to the center of one half.
3. Add the salmon inside.
4. Season with salt and pepper.
Almost spoonable like ice cream!!!

Parmesan Pizza

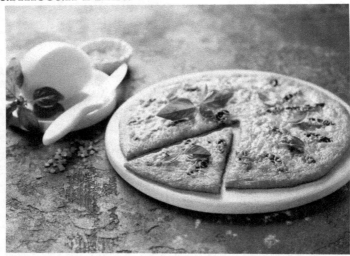

Ingredients for 1 portion:
- 2 tbsp parmesan
- 2 big eggs
- 2 cups tomato sauce
- 2 tbsp Evo oil
- 3 tbsp mozzarella cheese, cubed
- 1 tsp oregano
- 1 tsp basil
- Salt and pepper to taste

Nutrition 100 g:
Calories: 291 kcal
Fat: 12 g
Proteins: 24 g
Carbs: 2 g
Directions:
1. Use a blender to mix all the ingredients, eggs, parmesan, and spices, creating a sort of pizza-dough.
2. Heat the oil in a skillet, pour the mixture in. Once its edges are brown, flip and cook for 1-2 minutes.
3. Turn off and heat the grill. Add tomato sauce and cheese, then cook in the oven for 1-2 minutes, until cheese starts making bubbles. What a wonderful pizza!

Chicken Muffins

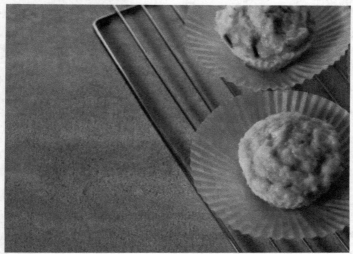

Ingredients for 2 portions:

- 2 tbsp mozzarella, diced
- 1 cup chicken, cooked and diced
- 1 egg
- 1 or 2 green peppers
- 1 tbsp fresh coriander
- Salt and pepper to taste

Nutrition 100 g:
Calories: 182 kcal
Fat: 8 g
Proteins: 28 g
Carbs: 3 g
Directions:
1. Preheat the oven at 300° F. Line some muffin molds with baking paper and set aside.
2. Cook the diced chicken with a little oil.
3. Beat the eggs together with green peppers, salt, pepper, mozzarella, and coriander in a bowl.
4. Pour the egg and chicken mixture into two muffin molds.
5. Bake for 10-15 minutes.
6. Let cool and serve.
What a meal!

Grandpa's Grilled Cheese

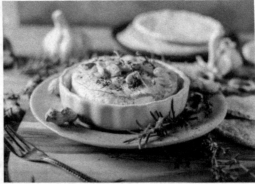

Ingredients for 1 portion:

- 4 tbsp Gorgonzola cheese (Taleggio or Brie are fine too)
- 2 tsp Evo oil
- 2 tsp minced walnuts
- 1 tsp fresh thyme, minced
- 1 pinch black pepper
- 1 tsp fresh parsley
- 1 garlic clove
- 1 pinch salt

Nutrition 100 g:
Calories: 362 kcal
Fat: 22 g
Proteins: 18 g
Carbs: 2 g
Directions:
1. Preheat the static oven at 400° F. Line a baking sheet with parchment paper.
2. In a bowl, mix the olive oil with the spices, parsley, garlic, thyme, rosemary, pepper, salt and chopped walnuts.
3. Mix well.
4. Lay the cheese on the baking paper and spread the herb and walnut mixture until the surface is covered.
5. Bake until cheese is soft and nuts are toasted.
They say feet can smell like cheese, but feet will no longer smell for you!

Viennese Chicken Wings

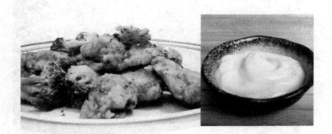

Ingredients for 1 portion:
- ½ cup broccoli
- 1 cup chicken wings
- 1 tbsp Evo oil
- 2 tbsp mayo, better if homemade
- 2 pinches of fresh dill
- 1 tsp minced or grated ginger
- 1 tsp red hot chili pepper, minced
- Salt and pepper to taste

Nutrition 100 g:
Calories: 212 kcal **Fat:** 14 g **Proteins:** 20 g **Carbs:** 2 g

Directions:
1. Prepare the marinade by mixing olive oil with salt, ground ginger and chili pepper.
2. Place the chicken wings in a sealable bag and add the prepared marinade.
3. Shake vigorously to coat wings evenly.
4. Preheat your oven to 400° F. Arrange the wings in a single layer in a greased baking dish. Bake for about 45 minutes.
5. While the chicken wings are in the oven, bring a pot of water to a boil and cook the broccoli.
6. Season the steamed broccoli with salt, fresh dill, black pepper, and mayonnaise. You can cream the broccoli with a blender.
7. Mix the cream with chicken until evenly seasoned.

Superfine recipe!

Flowering Mushrooms

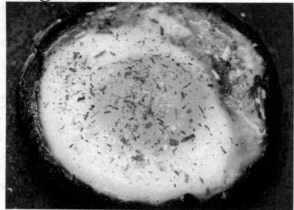

Ingredients for 1 portion:
- 3 tbsp grated parmesan
- 1 champignon mushroom, better if Portobello
- 1 egg
- 1 tbsp Evo oil
- ½ tsp thyme
- Salt and pepper to taste

Nutrition 100 g:
Calories: 194 kcal
Fat: 14 g
Proteins: 18 g
Carbs: 1 g
Directions:
1. Preheat the oven at 400° F.
2. In a baking dish, place the mushroom cap down and drizzle with olive oil.
3. Sprinkle with thyme and salt and place in the preheated oven to bake for 3-5 minutes.
4. Remove from oven. Sprinkle with grated parmesan cheese.
5. Crack an egg into the groove left by the Portobello stem, sprinkle with thyme and salt and return the mushroom to the oven.
6. Sprinkle with thyme and salt and return the mushrooms to the oven.
7. Bake for 8-10 minutes or until cooked through.
A dish for true connoisseurs!

Homemade Cheese

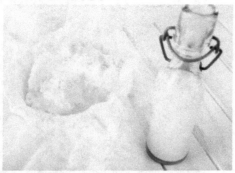

Ingredients for 1 mold:

- 1 l fresh milk
- 1 white or unsweetened Greek yogurt
- Juice ½ lemon
- A 40 inches cotton gauze (you can find it in any pharmacy)

Nutrition 100 g:
Calories: 272 kcal
Fat: 22 g
Proteins: 17 g
Carbs: 1 g
Directions:

1. Add the yogurt to the milk, pour everything in a saucepan and bring to pre-boil (180° F), then add lemon juice. Mix quickly, then let cool. You'll see the lumps (rennet) rising on the surface.

2. Divide the whey from the rennet, wrap it in the gauze and squeeze it. The rennet will remain on the gauze, while the whey will be poured into the bowl.

3. Squeeze the gauze tightly over the mass to drain the liquid as much as possible. Drain the whey from the bowl and place the gauze with the cheese inside. Squeeze once more, then place in the refrigerator for 1 night; place a weight (a jar, for example) on top of the bowl to obtain the round shape.

4. Open the gauze and sprinkle a pinch of salt. Compress the gauze around the cheese again and let it rest in the fridge for another 8 hours. After the waiting time has elapsed, you'll have prepared a delicious homemade cheese with a few simple and easily available ingredients! What a nice activity it's to make our own cheese!

Cheese and Walnuts Salad

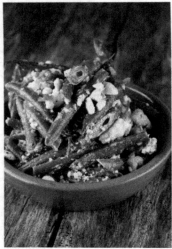

Ingredients for 1 portion:

- ½ cup green beans, cooked or canned
- ¼ cup cheese (Asiago, or whatever you like)
- 2 tbsp walnuts
- 4 tbsp carrots
- 2 cups avocado
- 2 tbsp Evo oil
- Salt and pepper to taste

Nutrition:

Calories: 454 kcal

Fat: 42 g

Carbs: 4 g

Proteins: 14 g

Directions:

1. Steam green beans (fresh, but canned are fine as well).

2. Cut cheese and avocado into cubes. Mince walnuts and cut carrots into strips.

3. Combine everything in a bowl. Season with oil, salt, and pepper.

A fresh and healthy salad!

Spiderman Salad

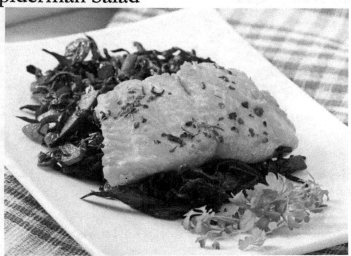

Ingredients for 1 portion:

- ½ cup smoked salmon
- ½ cup red cabbage
- 1 lemon
- 1 tsp gomasium
- 1 tbsp extra virgin olive oil
- Salt and pepper to taste

Nutrition for each portion:

Calories: 142 kcal

Carbs: 6 g

Fat: 16 g

Proteins: 10 g

Directions:

1. Cut some of the cabbage, wash it and slice it into thin strips. Place it in a bowl and drizzle with lemon juice and add a pinch of gomasium.

2. Let it marinate in the fridge for at least 2 hours. Serve with salmon strips and season with oil, spices, and the rest of gomasium.

Variation:

As an alternative to red cabbage, you can also use some arugula or radicchio or mixed salad.

You'll feel like Superman!

Genovese Squids

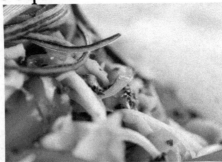

Ingredients for 4 portions:
- 3 and 1/3 cups fresh gutted or defrosted squid
- 2 cups carrots
- 2 and ½ cups zucchini (celery, fennel to taste)
- 2 tbsp radishes
- 1 spring fresh parsley
- 1 lemon
- Salt, pepper, and oregano to taste
- 4 tbsp extra virgin olive oil

Nutrition for 1 portion:
Calories: 205 kcal **Carbs:** 10 g **Fat:** 12 g **Proteins:** 20 g

Directions:
1. Gut fresh squid (or buy them down gutted from the fishmonger or thawed), separate the body from the tentacles and cut the body into rounds while reducing the tentacles into smaller pieces.
2. Wash the zucchini and dice them.
3. Boil the squid in a saucepan full of water for about 10 minutes from the moment it starts to boil.
4. About 3 minutes before the end of cooking, add the diced zucchini. Drain the squid and zucchini and let cool.
5. In the meantime, after washing the vegetables with soda baking, remove the outer skin from the carrots and grate them into cubes; cut the radishes into slices.
6. Squeeze the juice of 1 lemon and keep the grated peel aside.
7. Take a large bowl and start combining all the ingredients: the cooked squid and zucchinis, the carrots, and raw radishes. Season with lemon juice, grated peel, oregano, chopped parsley, salt, pepper, and oil. What a salad!

Turmeric Fennels

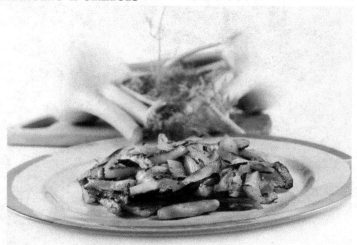

Ingredients for 4 portions:
- 6 cups fresh fennels
- 4 tbsp Evo oil
- 1 tbsp turmeric powder
- 1 tbsp almond flour
- Salt, mint leaves to taste

Nutrition for 1 portion:
Calories: 102 kcal
Carbs: 3 g
Fat: 10 g
Proteins: 2 g
Directions:
1. Wash the fennels and cut the head and bottom. Slice them vertically and place them on a baking pan, one next to the other.
2. Melt the turmeric in a ½ glass hot water and pour into the pan.
3. Sprinkle the surface with almond flour, salt, and mint leaves.
4. Cook in the oven for 20 minutes at 360° F. Grill them before serving.
Cooked vegetables are lighter!

Scottona Slices with Pumpkin

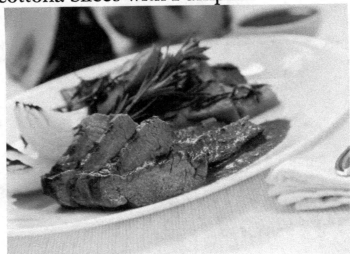

Ingredients for 2 portions:

- 10 ounces scottona, sliced (scottona or any other meat)
- 10 ounces pumpkin, cleaned
- 1 small shallot
- 4 tbsp Evo oil
- 1 tsp wild fennel seeds
- Salt and pepper to taste

Nutrition for 1 portion:

Calories: 297 kcal

Carbs: 6 g

Fat: 16 g

Proteins: 33 g

Directions:

1. Remove the outer skin from the pumpkin and slice it.

2. Take a non-stick pan and sauté the sliced shallot with the oil. Add meat, pumpkin, and salt.

3. Let it cook for 10 minutes, turning the slices on the other side as well. If they ended up being too dry, add some vegetable broth.

4. Sprinkle with ground black pepper and serve.

A truly delicious dish, don't you think?

Eggs with Tuna and Veggies

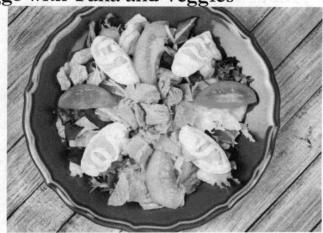

Ingredients for 4 portions:

- 8 eggs, hard-boiled, chopped
- 28 ounces (795 g) tuna in brine, drained
- 4 cup lettuces, torn into pieces
- ½ cup green onions, finely chopped
- ½ tablespoon mustard
- 2 tomatoes, diced
- Salt and pepper to taste

Nutritional values:
Calories: 186 Kcal
Fat: 8 g
Protein: 30 g
Carbs: 2 g
Directions:
1. Put the eggs on a plate. Add the tuna, onion, lettuce, tomatoes and mustard.

Chorizo, Kale, and Avocado Eggs

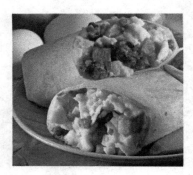

Ingredients for 2 portions:
- 1 teaspoon butter 1 red onion sliced
- 4 ounces (114 g) chorizo, sliced into thin rounds
- 1 cup chopped kale
- 1 ripe avocado, pitted, peeled, chopped
- 4 fresh eggs
- 2 low carb burritos
- Salt and black pepper to season

Nutritional values:
Calories: 305 Kcal **Fat:** 23 g **Protein:** 14 g **Carbs:** 7g

Directions:
1. Preheat oven to 370°F (188°C).
2. Melt butter in a cast iron pan over medium heat and sauté the onion for 2 minutes.
3. Add the chorizo and cook for 2 minutes more, flipping once.
4. Introduce the kale in batches with a splash of water to wilt, season lightly with salt, stir and cook for 3 minutes.
5. Mix in the avocado and turn the heat off.
6. Create four holes in the mixture, crack the eggs into each hole, sprinkle with salt and black pepper, and slide the pan into the preheated oven to bake for 6 minutes until the egg whites are set or firm and yolks still runny.
7. Season to taste with salt and pepper, and serve right away with low carb burrito.

Dill-Cream-Cheese Salmon Rolls

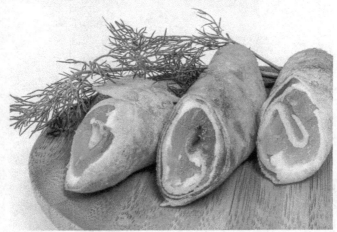

Ingredients for 3 portions:
- 3 tablespoons cream cheese, softened
- 1 lemon, zested and juiced
- 3 teaspoons chopped fresh dill
- Salt and black pepper to taste
- 3 (7-inch) low carb tortillas
- 6 slices smoked salmon

Nutritional values:
Calories: 251 Kcal
Fat: 16 g
Protein: 18 g
Carbs: 7 g

Directions:
1. In a bowl, mix the cream cheese, lemon juice, zest, dill, salt, and black pepper.
2. Lay each tortilla on a plastic wrap (just wide enough to cover the tortilla), spread with cream cheese mixture, and top each (one) with two salmon slices.
3. Roll up the tortillas and secure both ends by twisting.
4. Refrigerate for 2 hours, remove plastic, cut off both ends of each wrap, and cut wraps into wheels.

Cheese and Egg Spinach Nests

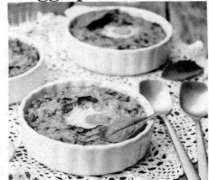

Ingredients for 4 portions:
- 2 tablespoons olive oil
- 1 clove garlic, grated
- ½ pound (227 g) spinach, chopped
- Salt and black pepper to taste
- 2 tablespoons shredded Parmesan cheese
- 2 tablespoons shredded gouda cheese
- 4 eggs
- 2 low carb toasts

Nutritional values:
Calories: 231 Kcal
Fat: 18 g
Protein: 13 g
Carbs: 4 g

Directions:
1. Preheat oven to 350°F (180°C).
2. Warm the oil in a non-stick skillet over medium heat; add the garlic and sauté until softened for 2 minutes.
3. Add the spinach to wilt for about 5 minutes, and season with salt and black pepper. Allow cooling.
4. Grease a baking sheet with cooking spray, mold 4 (firm and separate) spinach nests on the sheet, and crack an egg into each nest. Sprinkle with Parmesan and gouda cheese.
5. Bake for 15 minutes just until the egg whites have set and the yolks are still runny.
6. Plate the nests and serve right away with low carb toasts and coffee.

Mushroom and Broccoli Quiche

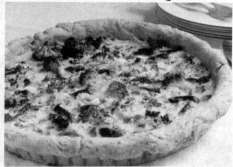

Ingredients for 6 portions:
- 12 eggs
- 2 cups shredded Cheddar cheese
- 1½ cups almond milk
- ½ teaspoon dried thyme
- ¼ cup chopped mushrooms, ½ cup chopped broccoli
- 1 clove garlic, minced and salt and black pepper to taste

Quiche Pastry:
- ¾ cup almond flour
- 2 ounces (58 g) cold butter
- ½ teaspoon baking powder
- 1 tablespoon cold water
- 2 eggs

Nutritional values:
Calories: 477 Kcal **Fat:** 40 g
Protein: 25 g **Carbs:** 6 g
Directions:
1. Preheat the oven to 370°F (188°C).
2. In a large bowl, mix all the crust ingredients until dough is formed.
3. Press it into a greased baking dish and bake for 20-25 minutes until lightly golden.
4. Spread the Cheddar cheese in the pie crust. Beat the eggs with the almond milk, thyme, salt and pepper, then, stir in the mushrooms, broccoli, and garlic. Pour the ingredients into the pie crust and bake in the oven for 35 minutes until the quiche is set.

Tomato and Bacon Cups

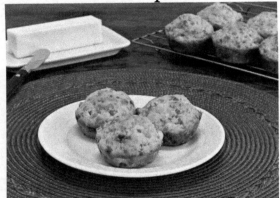

Ingredients for 6 portions:

- 12 bacon slices
- 2 tomatoes, diced
- 1 onion, diced
- 1 cup shredded Cheddar cheese
- 1 cup mayonnaise
- 12 low carb crepes/pancakes
- 1 teaspoon dried basil

Nutritional values:
Calories: 426 Kcal
Fat: 45 g
Protein: 16 g
Carbs: 5 g
Directions:
1. Fry the bacon in a skillet over medium heat for 5 minutes.
2. Remove and chop with a knife.
3. Transfer to a bowl. Add in Cheddar cheese, tomatoes, onion, mayonnaise, and basil. Mix well set aside.
4. Place the crepes on a flat surface and use egg rings to cut a circle out of each crepe.
5. Grease the muffin cups with cooking spray and fit the circled crepes into them to make a cup.
6. Now, fill the cups with 3 tablespoons of bacon-tomato mixture. Place the muffin cups on a baking sheet, and bake for 18 minutes.

Triple Cheese and Bacon Zucchini Balls

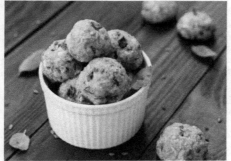

Ingredients for 4 portions:
- 4 cups zucchini, spiralized
- ½ pound (228 g) bacon, chopped and 1 cup crushed pork rinds
- 6 ounces (170 g) cottage cheese, curds and 6 ounces (170 g) cream cheese
- 1 cup Fontina cheese ½ cup dill pickles, chopped, squeezed and 1 cup grated Parmesan cheese
- 2 cloves garlic, crushed
- ½ teaspoon caraway seeds
- ¼ teaspoon dried dill weed
- ½ teaspoon onion powder
- Cooking oil, salt and black pepper, to taste
- Fresh parsley and mayo to garnish

Nutritional values:
Calories: 406 Kcal Fat: 27 g Protein: 33 g **Carbs:** 5 g

Directions:
1. Thoroughly mix zoodles, cottage cheese, dill pickles, ½ cup of Parmesan cheese, garlic, cream cheese, bacon, and Fontina cheese until well combined. Shape the mixture into balls. Refrigerate for 3 hours.

2. In a mixing bowl, mix the remaining ½ cup of Parmesan cheese, crushed pork rinds, dill, black pepper, onion powder, caraway seeds, and salt. Roll cheese ball in Parmesan mixture to coat.

3. Set a skillet over medium heat and warm 1-inch of oil. Fry cheeseballs until browned on all sides.

4. Set on a paper towel to soak up any excess oil.

Peppery Omelet with Cheddar Cheese

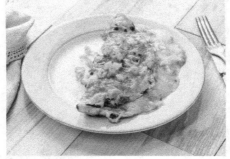

Ingredients for 2 portions:
- 2 tablespoons olive oil
- 1 onion sliced
- 2 bell peppers chopped
- 1 jalapeño pepper chopped
- 4 eggs whisked
- 4 tablespoons full-fat yogurt
- sea salt
- ground black pepper
- 3 ounces (85 g) Cheddar cheese shredded
- Red pepper and chopped green onions to garnish

Nutritional values:
Calories: 439 Kcal
Fat: 37 g
Protein: 23 g
Carbs: 4 g

Directions:
1. Heat the olive oil in a frying pan over a moderate flame.
2. Sauté the onion and peppers for 3 minutes, until tender and fragrant.
3. Then, mix the eggs with the full-fat yogurt. Now, pour the egg mixture into the frying pan. Season with salt and black pepper.
4. Move the pan around to spread it out evenly. Continue to cook for about 5 minutes until the eggs are fully set and the surface is smooth.
5. Top with cheese and serve immediately.

Broccoli and Ham Egg Bake

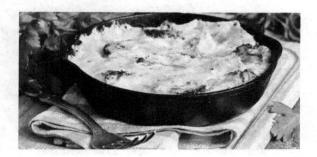

Ingredients for 4 portions:
- 2 heads broccoli, cut into small florets
- 2 red bell peppers, seeded and chopped
- ¼ cup chopped ham
- 2 teaspoons butter
- 1 teaspoon dried oregano plus extra to garnish
- Salt, black pepper and oregano to taste
- 8 fresh eggs

Nutritional values:
Calories: 345 Kcal
Fat: 28 g
Protein: 11 g **Carbs:** 4 g
Directions:
1. Preheat oven to 425°F (220°C).
2. Melt the butter in a frying pan over medium heat; brown the ham, stirring frequently, about 3 minutes.
3. Arrange the broccoli, bell peppers, and ham on a foil-lined baking sheet in a single layer, toss to combine; season with salt, oregano, and black pepper.
4. Bake for 10 minutes until the vegetables have softened. 5. Remove, create eight indentations with a spoon, and crack an egg into each.
5. Return to the oven and continue to bake for an additional 5 to 7 minutes until the egg whites are firm. Season with salt, black pepper, and extra oregano, share the bake into four plates.

Avocado Sausage Stacks

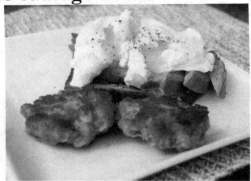

Ingredients for 6 portions:
- 6 Italian sausage patties
- 4 tablespoons olive oil
- 2 ripe avocados, pitted
- 2 teaspoons fresh lime juice
- Salt, black pepper
- 6 fresh eggs
- Red pepper flakes to garnish

Nutritional values:
Calories: 388 Kcal **Fat:** 23 g **Protein:** 16 g **Carbs:** 9 g

Directions:
1. In a skillet, warm the oil over medium heat and fry the sausage patties about 8 minutes until lightly browned and firm.
2. Remove the patties to a plate.
3. Spoon the avocado into a bowl, mash with the lime juice, and season with salt and black pepper.
4. Spread the mash on the sausages.
5. Boil 3 cups of water in a wide pan over high heat, and reduce to simmer.
6. Crack each egg into a small bowl and gently put the egg into the simmering water; poach for 2 to 3 minutes. Use a perforated spoon to remove from the water on a paper towel to dry.
7. Repeat with the other 5 eggs.
8. Top each stack with a poached egg, sprinkle with chili flakes, salt, black pepper, and chives.
9. Plate, and serve with low carb crusted bread.

Mushroom and Kale Tofu Scramble

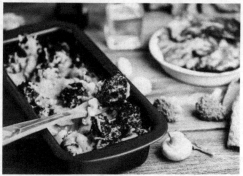

Ingredients for 4 portions:
- 2 tablespoons butter ghee
- 1 cup sliced white mushrooms
- 2 cloves garlic, minced
- 16 ounces (455 g) firm tofu, pressed and crumbled
- Salt and black pepper to taste
- 1 cup thinly sliced kale
- 6 fresh eggs

Nutritional values:
Calories: 470 Kcal
Fat: 38 g
Protein: 25 g
Carbs: 5 g

Directions:
1. Melt the butter in a non-stick skillet over medium heat, and sauté the mushrooms for 5 minutes until they lose their liquid.
2. Add the garlic and cook for 1 minute.
3. Crumble the tofu into the skillet, season with salt and black pepper. Cook with continuous stirring for 6 minutes.
4. Introduce the kale in batches and cook to soften for about 7 minutes.
5. Crack the eggs into a bowl, whisk until well combined and creamy in color, and pour all over the kale.
6. Use a spatula to immediately stir the eggs while cooking until scrambled and no more runny, about 5 minutes.
7. Plate, and serve with low carb crusted bread.

Cream Cheese Almond Muffins

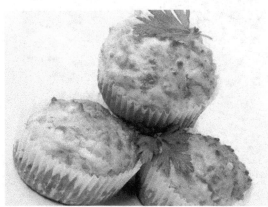

Ingredients for 4 portions:
- 2 drops liquid stevia
- 2 cups almond flour
- 2 teaspoons baking powder
- ½ teaspoon salt
- 8 ounces (227 g) cream cheese, softened
- ¼ cup melted butter
- 1 egg
- 1 cup unsweetened almond milk

Nutritional values:
Calories: 321 Kcal
Fat: 30 g
Protein: 5 g
Carbs: 5 g

Directions:
1. Preheat oven to 400°F (205°C) and grease a 12-cup muffin tray with cooking spray.
2. Mix the flour, baking powder, and salt in a large bowl. In a separate bowl, beat the cream cheese, stevia, and butter using a hand mixer and whisk in the egg and milk.
3. Fold in the flour, and spoon the batter into the muffin cups two-thirds way up.
4. Bake for 20 minutes until puffy at the top and golden brown, remove to a wire rack to cool slightly for 5 minutes before serving.

Swiss Chard, Sausage, and Squash Omelet

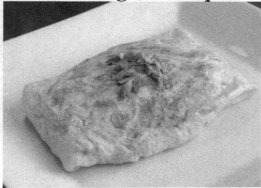

Ingredients for 1 portion:
- 2 eggs
- 1 cup Swiss chard, chopped
- 4 ounces (114 g) sausage, chopped
- 2 tablespoons ricotta cheese
- 4 ounces (114 g) roasted squash
- 1 tablespoon olive oil
- Salt and black pepper, to taste
- Fresh parsley to garnish

Nutritional values:
Calories: 550 Kcal **Fat:** 50 g **Protein:** 32 g Carbs: 7 g

Directions:
1. Beat the eggs in a bowl, season with salt and pepper; stir in the Swiss chard and the ricotta cheese.
2. In another bowl, mash the squash and add to the egg mixture.
3. Heat ¼ tablespoon of olive oil in a pan over medium heat. Add sausage and cook until browned on all sides, turning occasionally. Drizzle the remaining olive oil.
4. Pour the egg mixture over. Cook for about 2 minutes per side until the eggs are thoroughly cooked and lightly browned.
5. Remove the pan and run a spatula around the edges of the omelet; slide it onto a warm platter. Fold in half, and serve sprinkled with fresh parsley.

Sausage Quiche

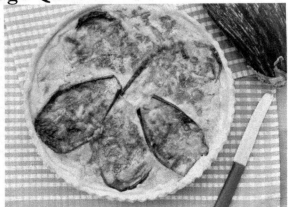

Ingredients for 6 portions:
- 6 eggs
- 12 ounces (340 g) raw sausage roll
- 10 cherry tomatoes, halved
- 2 tablespoons heavy cream
- 2 tablespoons Parmesan cheese
- ¼ teaspoon salt
- A pinch of black pepper
- 5 eggplant slices
- Lettuce to garnish

Nutritional values:
Calories: 337 Kcal
Fat: 28 g
Protein: 18 g
Carbs: 3 g

Directions:
1. Preheat your oven to 370°F (188°C). Grease a pie dish with cooking spray.
2. Press the sausage roll at the bottom of a pie dish.
3. Arrange the eggplant slices on top of the sausage. Top with cherry tomatoes.
4. Whisk the eggs along with the heavy cream, salt, Parmesan cheese, and black pepper. Spoon the mixture over the sausage.
5. Bake for about 40 minutes until browned around the edges.
6. Serve warm, sprinkled with parsley.

Gruyere and Mushroom Lettuce Wraps

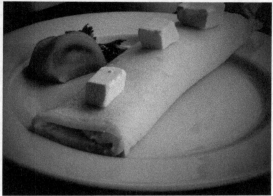

Ingredients for 4 portions:
Wraps:

- 6 eggs - 2 tablespoons almond milk
- 1 tablespoon olive oil and sea salt, to taste

Filling:

- 1 teaspoon olive oil
- 1 cup mushrooms, chopped
- Salt and black pepper, to taste
- ½ teaspoon cayenne pepper
- 8 fresh lettuce leaves
- 4 slices Gruyere cheese
- 2 tomatoes, sliced

Nutritional values:
Calories: 477 Kcal **Fat:** 44 g **Protein:** 20 g **Carbs:** 5 g
Directions:
1. Mix all the ingredients for the wraps thoroughly.
2. Set a frying pan over medium heat. Add in ¼ of the mixture and cook for 4 minutes on both sides.
3. Do the same thrice and set the wraps aside, they should be kept warm.
4. In a separate pan over medium heat, warm 1 teaspoon of olive oil. Cook the mushrooms for 5 minutes until soft; add cayenne pepper, black pepper, and salt.
5. Set 1-2 lettuce leaves onto every wrap, split the mushrooms among the wraps and top with tomatoes and cheese.

Bacon and Zucchini Hash

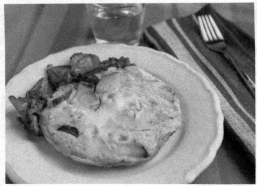

Ingredients for 1 portion:
- 1 medium zucchini, diced
- 2 bacon slices
- 2 egg
- 1 tablespoon coconut oil
- ½ small onion, chopped
- 1 tablespoon chopped parsley
- ¼ teaspoon salt
- 2 slices Cheddar cheese

Nutritional values:
Calories: 381 Kcal
Fat: 32 g
Protein: 20 g
Carbs: 6 g

Directions:
1. Place the bacon in a skillet and cook for a few minutes, until crispy. Remove and set aside.
2. Warm the coconut oil and cook the onion until soft, for about 3-4 minutes, occasionally stirring. Add the zucchini, and cook for 10 more minutes until zucchini is brown and tender, but not mushy.
3. Transfer to a plate and season with salt.
4. Crack the eggs into the same skillet and fry over medium heat. Top the zucchini mixture with the bacon slices, cheese and a fried eggs.

Feta Spinach Frittata

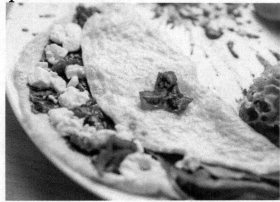

Ingredients for 4 portions:
- 5 ounces (143 g) spinach
- 8 ounces (228 g) crumbled Feta cheese
- 1 pint halved cherry tomatoes
- 10 eggs
- 3 tablespoons olive oil
- 4 scallions, diced
- Salt and black pepper, to taste

Nutrition 100 g:
Calories: 242 kcal
Fat: 22 g
Proteins: 24 g
Carbs: 3 g
Directions:
1. Preheat your oven to 350°F (180°C).
2. Drizzle the oil in a casserole and place in the oven until heated.
3. In a bowl, whisk the eggs along with the black pepper and salt, until thoroughly combined. Stir in the spinach, Feta cheese, and scallions.
4. Pour the mixture into the casserole, top with the cherry tomatoes and place back in the oven. Bake for 25 minutes until your frittata is set in the middle.
5. When done, remove the casserole from the oven and run a spatula around the edges of the frittata; slide it onto a warm platter and cut the frittata into wedges.

Chapter 3
Smoothies

Chocolate Smoothie in the Woods

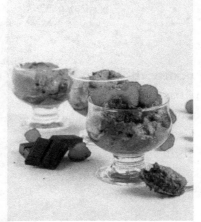

Ingredients for 1 portion:
- 1/2 cup berries
- 1 cup coconut cream
- 1 tbsp coconut oil
- 1/4 cup cacao powder
- 1 tbsp erythritol

Nutrition 100 g:
Calories: 354 kcal
Carbs: 8 g
Fat: 29 g
Proteins: 11 g
Directions:
1. Combine all the ingredients in a blender and mix.
2. Mix until you get a very creamy consistency.
Cheers!

St. Claus' Smoothie

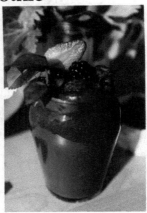

Ingredients for 1 portion:

- 1/2 cup berries
- 1 cup coconut cream
- 1/4 cup cocoa powder
- 1 tbsp erythritol

Nutrition 100 g:

Calories: 254 kcal

Carbs: 7 g

Fat: 25 g

Proteins: 11 g

Directions:

1. Add all the ingredients in a blender and mix quickly. And jump on St. Claus' sleigh!

Superman Smoothie

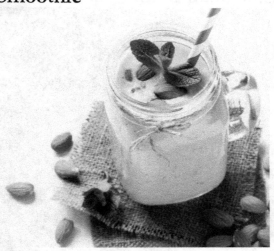

Ingredients for 1 portion:
- 3/4 cup almond milk, without sugars
- 1/4 cup coconut milk
- 1 tbsp almond butter and 1 tbsp coconut oil
- 1 tbsp vegetable protein powder

Nutrition 100 g:
Calories: 470 kcal
Carbs: 5 g
Proteins: 28 g
Fat: 38 g
Directions:
1. Combine all the ingredients in a blender. Serve and enjoy it.

Chocolate Bomb

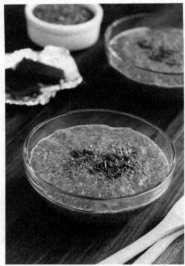

Ingredients for 1 portion:
- 1/2 cup coconut milk
- 1/2 cup hemp seeds
- 3 tsp clarified butter
- 1 tbsp chia seeds
- 2 tbsp cocoa powder
- 1 tsp erythritol
- ½ tsp vanilla extract
- 1 tsp coconut oil

Nutrition 100 g:
Calories: 287 kcal
Carbs: 5 g
Proteins: 14 g
Fat: 24 g

Directions:
1. Combine all the ingredients in a saucepan over low heat for 4-5 minutes.
2. Mix well until you get a homogeneous mixture. Pour in a cup and let it cool in the refrigerator for the whole night.
Finger-licking!

Wood Pudding

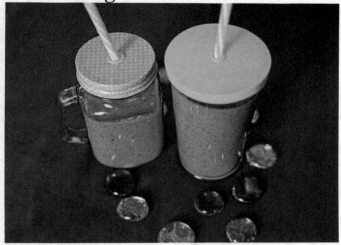

Ingredients for 2 portions:

- 1 cup coconut oil
- 1 cup fresh raspberries
- 2 tsp coconut oil
- 1 tbsp apple vinegar
- 1 tsp vanilla extract
- 1 tsp erythritol
- 2 tbsp chia seeds
- 1 tsp sesame seeds

Nutrition for 1 portion:

Calories: 218 kcal

Carbs: 7 g

Proteins: 7 g

Fat: 19 g

Directions:

1. Combine all the ingredients in a blender, mix everything.
2. Serve cold.

Dreamy!

Fit Smoothie

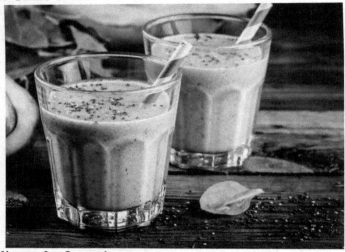

Ingredients for 2 portions:

- 1 and ½ cup almond milk
- 1 cup spinach
- 1 cucumber
- 1 celery
- 1 courgette
- 1 Avocado
- 1 tbsp coconut oil
- 2 tsp erythritol
- 1 tbsp protein powder
- 1 tsp chia seeds

Nutrition for each portion:
Calories: 120 kcal
Carbs: 3 g
Proteins: 21 g
Fat: 16 g
Directions:
1. Put the spinach first in a blender, then add the almond milk.
2. Mix the other ingredients, except for the chia seeds.
3. Serve garnishing with chia seeds.
And you'll be fit!

Hot Chocolate in a Cup

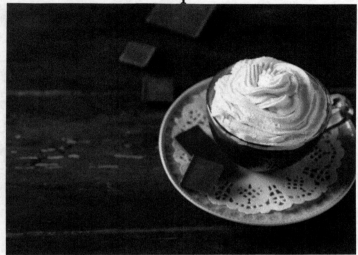

Ingredients for 1 portion:
- 2 tbsp cocoa powder
- 1 tbsp clarified butter
- 2 tbsp whole cream for desserts
- 1 tsp vanilla extract
- 1 tsp erythritol

Nutrition for each portion:
Calories: 134 kcal
Carbs: 2 g
Proteins: 6 g
Fat: 12 g

Directions:
1. In a blender, mix the ingredients.
2. Add cacao powder.
3. Add butter and the vanilla extract and mix with a cup of hot water until you get a creamy and homogeneous mixture.
4. Pour in a cup and garnish with the whole cream.
Enjoy your hot chocolate!

Shaked Cold Coffee

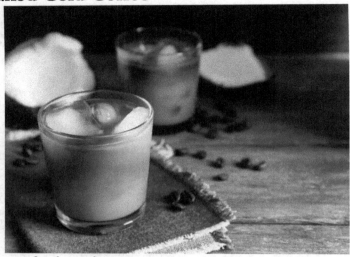

Ingredients for 1 portion:
- 1 tsp clarified butter
- 1 cup freshly brewed coffee
- 2 tbsp coconut oil
- 2-3 ice cubes
- 1 tsp erythritol (if you want it sweet)

Nutrition:

Calories: 124 kcal

Carbs: 0 g

Proteins: 0 g

Fat: 14 g

Directions:

1. Combine all the ingredients in a blender without ice.

2. Mix until you get a homogeneous and creamy mixture.

3. Add ice and mix for another 15-20 minutes.

4. Serve immediately.

Coffee is yummier during summer!

Batman Cocktail

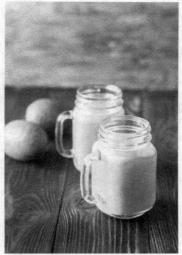

Ingredients for 1 portion:
- 3 tbsp coconut cream
- 1 tbsp coconut oil
- 1 cup frozen spinach
- Juice from 1 lemon (or lime)
- 2 tsp grated ginger, fresh
- ½ cup water

Nutrition for 1 portion:
Calories: 103 kcal
Carbs: 3 g
Proteins: 1 g
Fat: 10 g
Directions:
1. Put the spinach in a blender.
2. Add fresh ginger and coconut oil.
3. Add coconut cream and water.
4. Blend until you get a homogeneous mix.
Your voice is going to become as gravelly as Batman's!

Vegetable Smoothie

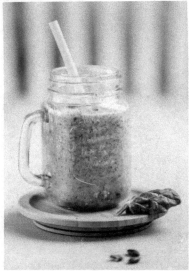

Ingredients:

- 2 cups spinach
- ½ cup coconut milk
- ½ cucumber
- 1 tsp erythritol
- 1 tbsp coconut oil
- 3 ice cubes

Nutrition for 1 portion:
Calories: 98 kcal
Carbs: 2 g
Proteins: 5 g
Fat: 9 g
Directions:
1. Put the spinaches in a blender, add the 3 ice cubes, coconut milk, erythritol and coconut oil.
2. Peel the cucumber and cube it, adding it to the mixer.
3. Blend the mixture for 1-2 minutes or until all the ingredients will be very well incorporated.
Amazing for your wellness!

Superman Shake

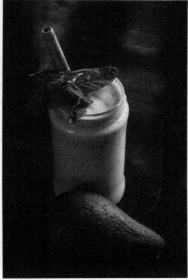

Ingredients for 4 portions:
- 3 cups flax milk, chilled
- 1 medium avocado, pitted, peeled, sliced
- 1 cup coconut milk, chilled
- 3 mint leaves plus extra to garnish
- 3 tablespoons erythritol
- 1 tablespoon low carb Protein powder

Nutritional values:
Calories: 266 Kcal
Fat: 16 g
Protein: 12 g
Carbs: 4 g

Directions:
1. Combine flax milk, avocado, coconut milk, 3 mint leaves, erythritol and protein powder in the smoothie maker and blend for 1 minute to make a smooth blend.
2. Pour the drink into serving glasses and garnish with 2 mint leaves.

Almond Shake

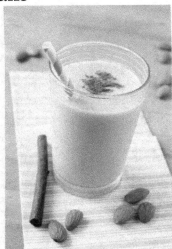

Ingredients for 1 portion:
- 1½ cups almond milk
- 2 tablespoons almond butter
- ½ teaspoon almond extract
- ½ teaspoon cinnamon
- 2 tablespoons flax meal
- 1 tablespoon collagen peptides
- A pinch of salt
- 15 drops of stevia
- A handful of ice cubes
- Cinnamon to taste

Nutritional values:
Calories: 327 Kcal **Fat:** 27 g **Protein:** 20 g **Carbs:** 6 g

Directions:
1. Add almond milk, almond butter, flax meal, almond extract, collagen peptides, a pinch of salt, and stevia to the bowl of a blender.
2. Blitz until uniform and smooth, for about 30 seconds.
3. Add a bit more almond milk if it's very thick. Then taste, and adjust flavor as needed, adding more stevia for sweetness or almond butter to the creaminess.
4. Pour in a smoothie glass, add the ice cubes and sprinkle with cinnamon.

Chapter 4
Dessert

Chocolate Cake

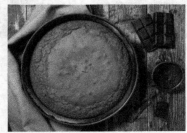

Ingredients for 6 portions:
- 1/4 cup chocolate (85% cocoa)
- 1/3 ghee or clarified butter
- 3 eggs - Salt to taste
- Vanilla extract to taste
- Coconut oil to grease the pan

Nutrition for 1 portion:
Calories: 241 kcal **Fat:** 21 g **Proteins:** 4 g **Carbs:** 8 g
Directions:
Preheat the oven at 380° F. Use a baking pan with a maximum 7 inches diameter. Grease the pan with coconut oil and secure a round piece of baking paper to the bottom. Break the chocolate into pieces and dice the butter. Melt them together in a double boiler or microwave. Be careful: Stir gently or the chocolate will burn. Once you have a smooth mixture, let it cool. Separate the yolks and egg whites and place them in separate bowls. Add salt to egg whites and beat with a mixer until whipped. Set aside. Add vanilla to egg yolks and beat until smooth. Add the melted chocolate and butter mixture to the egg yolks and mix well. Incorporate the beaten egg whites and mix well. Pour the mixture into the pan and bake for about 20-25 minutes, checking the degree of cooking with a toothpick. If you want, you can add a bit of whipped cream without sugar or some berries. Finger-licking!

Berries Cheesecake

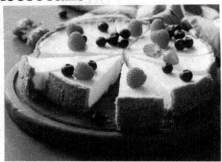

Ingredients for 6 portions:
Base:

- ½ cup almond flour - ¼ clarified butter
- 2 tbsp erythritol - ¼ tsp vanilla extract
- 1 tsp xanthan

Filling:

- 1 and ¼ cup Philadelphia or cream cheese
- 100 ml whipping cream without sugar
- 1 egg- ½ egg white
- 1 tbsp erythritol - Grated lemon zest to taste
- ¼ tsp vanilla extract - ¼ cup fresh blueberries

Nutrition 100 g:
Calories: 333 kcal **Fat:** 32 g **Proteins:** 7 g **Carbs:** 4 g

Directions:

1. Preheat the oven at 380° F.

2. Butter a small cake pan about 4 inches and line the base with baking paper. Melt the butter for the base and heat it for a few minutes. Remove from heat and add the almond flour, sweetener, and vanilla. Combine everything into a dough to place in the base of the cake pan. Bake for 8 minutes until the base turns slightly golden.

3. Set aside and let cool. Meanwhile, mix the cheese, cream, eggs, lemon zest, vanilla, and sweetener. Pour the mixture over the base.

9. Raise the oven temperature at 400° F and bake for 15 minutes, then lower it to 220° F and bake for another 45-60 minutes.

10. Turn off the oven and let the cake cool inside.

11. Remove it when it's completely cooled and put it in the refrigerator to rest overnight. When serving, add berries. You'll be in paradise!

Mom's Mascarpone

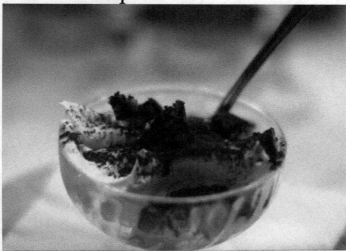

Ingredients for 2 portions:
- 4 egg yolks
- 10 gr erythritol or 20 gr, based on how sweet you want it

Nutrition 100 g:
Calories: 133 kcal
Fat: 6 g
Proteins: 25 g
Carbs: 0 g
Directions:
1. Place the four egg yolks in a bowl (if possible, make sure it's made of glass), add the erythritol and mix with a hand or electric whisk until creamy.
2. Pour into a champagne glass type glass, let sit in the fridge for an hour if possible. If you really want it that badly, then eat it right away!
P.S. you can also add dark chocolate chips without sugar.
This is how you taste heaven!

Explosive Cake

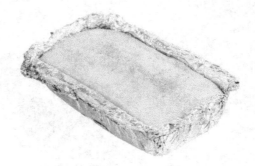

Ingredients:
- 2 cups almond flour
- 1/3 cup almond, minced
- ½ cup almond, whole
- 1/3 cup hazelnuts, whole
- 1 cup egg whites
- 1/3 cup erythritol
- 1 sachet instant yeast
- 1 tbsp xanthan

Glazing:
- ¼ cup peanut butter
- 50 gr Kefir
- Dried fruits

Nutrition 100 g:
Calories: 580 kcal **Fat:** 50 g **Proteins:** 21 g **Carbs:** 6 g
Directions:
1. Combine yeats and erythritol in a bowl, then add egg whites and mix until you get a homogeneous and creamy mix.
2. Add dried fruits and bake for 30 minutes at 380° F. Then pour the glaze.
Glazing:
Combine and mix butter and Kefir, getting a dense mixture you'll spread on the surface. Place again in the oven for another 5 minutes. Both kids and grownups will love it!

Lemon Cake

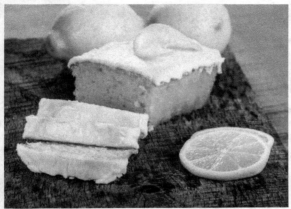

Ingredients for 1 portion:
- 1 egg - ¼ cup coconut flour
- 20 ml whole milk
- 1 tbsp clarified butter and 1 tbsp lemon juice
- 1 tbsp erythritol - ½ tsp baking powder
- Lemon zest and Salt to taste
- 1 tsp xanthan

Glazing:
- 2 tbsp creamy cheese - 1 tsp erythritol
- ¼ tsp vanilla extract - Lemon zest to taste

Nutrition 100 g:
Calories: 363 kcal **Fat:** 35 g **Proteins:** 12 g **Carbs:** 2 g
Directions:
1. Preheat your oven at 380° F.
2. Separate the egg whites from the yolks and beat the egg whites until stiff.
3. Add egg yolk, melted butter, coconut flour, erythritol, lemon juice, lemon zest, salt, and xanthan gum, and mix until smooth.
4. Butter a baking dish and pour in the mixture.
5. Bake in the oven for 45 to 50 minutes.
Glazing:
Mix the cream cheese with the erythritol powder, vanilla, and lemon zest.
Let the cake cool for 20 minutes and then top it with the frosting.
Volare oh oh, cantare oh oh oh!

Dreamy Pancakes

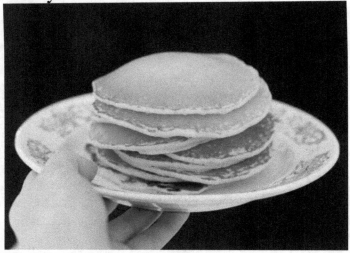

Ingredients for 3 portions:

- 4 eggs
- 1 tbsp melted butter
- 1/2 tsp cinnamon
- ¼ cup cream cheese
- ½ cup almond flour

Nutrition 100 g:
Calories: 370 kcal
Carbs: 5 g
Proteins: 24 g
Fat: 36 g
Directions:
1. Start by adding the ingredients to a blender and mix everything, except for the butter.
2. Heat a skillet over medium heat and melt the butter. Add 3 tbsp at a time of the mixture you've previously made, creating small pancakes.
3. Cook each side for 2 minutes.
All kids' dream!

Lemon Pie

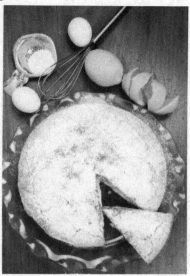

Ingredients:
- 1 cup almond flour
- 4 eggs
- 60 g Erythritol (mince it with a food processor)
- 1 lemon zest, grated
- 1 tsp xanthan powder
- 1 tsp psyllium powder

Nutrition for 1 portion:
Calories: 229 kcal
Carbs: 2 g
Proteins: 10 g
Fat: 18 g
Directions:
1. Whip the egg whites, beat the egg yolks with erythritol.
2. Add flour, grated lemon and psyllium to the yolks and gradually pour the egg whites.
3. Place in a baking pan and bake for 30 minutes at 360° F.
4. When it's ready, sprinkle erythritol on top.
You'll see angels after eating it!

Coffee and Walnuts Cake

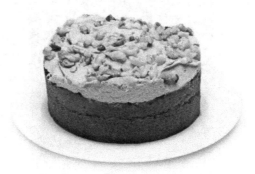

Ingredients for the cake itself:
- ¼ cup almond flour
- 1 cup walnuts, finely chopped
- 1 cup erythritol
- ½ clarified butter, melted
- 3 eggs
- 4 tsp coffee
- 1 tbsp xanthan

For the filling:
- 1 cup soft butter
- ½ cup erythritol powder
- 4 tsp coffee

Nutrition 100 g:
Calories: 470 kcal
Carbs: 5 g
Proteins: 18 gr
Fat: 30 gr

Directions:
1. Place the flour, walnuts, erythritol, butter in a bowl with eggs and coffee. Mix well with a mixer until well blended.
2. Roll out the flour mixture in a baking dish and place in a 350° F ventilated oven for 20 minutes.
3. Meanwhile, put the soft butter with the erythritol and coffee in another bowl. Mix well with a mixer. The filling mousse is ready.
4. Remove the cake from the oven and lay it cold on a plate. Spread the coffee mousse on top. Voilà! Satisfaction is served!

Artichoke Herbal Tea

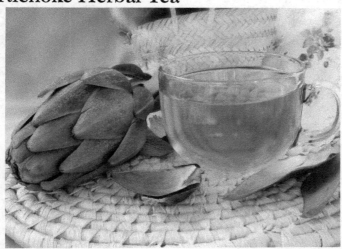

Ingredients for 2 liters:
- 3 artichokes

Nutrition for 1 cup:

Calories: 0 kcal

Carbs: 0 g

Proteins: 0 gr

Fat: 0 gr

Directions:

1. Clean the artichokes, cut off the part with thorns, steams and external leaves.

2. Dip the leaves in water and bring them to a boil.

3. Filter your prep after 20 minutes, keep in the fridge in a bottle made of glass. A real treat!

Superman's Sorbet

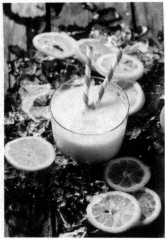

Ingredients:
- 1 cup fresh cream
- 2 tbsp erythritol
- Juice from 2 lemons

Nutrition 100 g:
Calories: 221 kcal
Carbs: 4 g
Proteins: 3 g
Fat: g
Directions:
1. Put the lemon juice in a bowl and pour erythritol and cream.
2. Blend well for 1 minute, then place in the freezer. If you want to get a mousse, blend for another 2 minutes.

Paradisiac Ice-cream

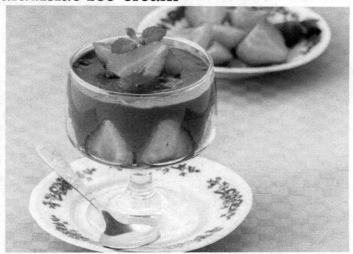

Ingredients:
- 2 cups whipping cream
- 1 tbsp cacao powder
- ½ cup erythritol

Nutrition 100 g:
Calories: 231 kcal
Carbs: 4 g
Proteins: 3 g
Fat: 35 g
Directions:
1. Place everything in a bowl and whip with a blender until you get a mousse.
2. Let it cool in the fridge for 4-5 hours before you eat it.
3. You can also add strawberries, hazelnuts, or a banana.
And you'll be heading towards paradise!

Japanese Cotton Cheesecake

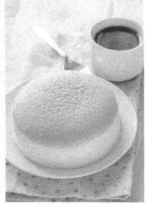

Ingredients:

- ½ cup almond flour
- 20 g Bamboo fiber/flour

Bamboo fiber/flour is important since it replaces potato starch. You can replace it also with coconut flour, but the consistency won't be the same.

- 3 eggs
- ½ cup Philadelphia
- ½ cup vegetal milk
- ¼ clarified butter
- ½ cup erythritol
- 2 tbsp lemon juice
- 1/2 lemon zest

Nutrition 100 g:

Calories: 591 kcal **Carbs:** 5 g **Proteins:** 23 g **Fat:** 50 g

Directions:

1. Separate yolks from egg whites and whip the latter until stiff.

2. Mix the cheese with softened butter, egg yolks and erythritol.

3. Add lemon juice and zest until well blended. Gently add the egg whites.

4. Bake in a 7 inches baking dish at about 360° F for 50 minutes without opening the oven.

5. Turn off the oven and leave the pan still inside to cool. Once cooled, keep the mixture in the refrigerator for a few hours. After, garnish as you wish. A Japanese smile will come out of your mouth!

Vanilla Cake

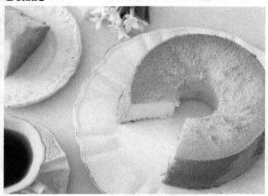

Ingredients:
- 1 egg
- 1 tbsp coconut oil
- 1 tsp vanilla extract
- 1 tbsp erythritol
- ½ cup almond milk
- 2 tbsp almond flour (or coconut flour)
- ½ tsp baking powder
- 1 pinch salt

Nutrition 100 g:
Calories: 131 kcal
Carbs: 3 g
Proteins: 8 g
Fat: 10 g
Directions:
1. In a bowl, add the almond milk and vanilla extract, mixing well.
2. Add the coconut oil and almond flour. Stir well.
3. Add the egg, erythritol and baking powder.
4. Mix until everything's combined.
5. Transfer the mixture to a microwaveable dish. Cook in a microwave for 90 to 120 seconds until it sets.
6. Or place in a preheated ventilated oven at 360° F for 45 minutes until the cake's fully cooked and you've done the toothpick test.
7. Let cool and serve.
Doesn't it remind you of your grandma?

Coconut and Strawberries Sorbet

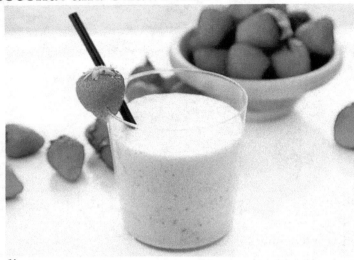

Ingredients:
- 3 tbsp coconut cream
- 1 tbsp fresh strawberries
- 1 tbsp coconut oil
- 1 tsp vanilla extract
- 3 cubed ice, chopped

Nutrition 100 g:
Calories: 112 kcal
Carbs: 5 g
Proteins: 6 g
Fat: 9 g
Directions:
1. Put the strawberries in a blender after washing them with soda. Add vanilla extracts and coconut oil.
2. Add coconut cream and add chopped ice. Blend until you get a homogeneous and creamy mixture.
Let it cool in the fridge for 1 hour.
A gentlemen's last course!

Chocolate and Avocado Pudding

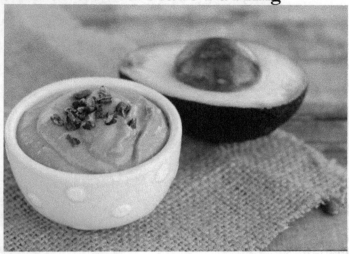

Ingredients:
- ½ avocado, mature and soft
- 1 tsp erythritol
- 3 tbsp cocoa powder
- 1 tsp vanilla extract

Nutrition 100 g:
Calories: 145 kcal
Carbs: 5 g
Proteins: 6 g
Fat: 9 g
Directions:
1. Remove the seed from the avocado and place the fruit in a bowl.
2. Add the cocoa powder, erythritol, and vanilla extract and mix with a fork until you get a creamy consistency. You can also use a blender for a few seconds.
3. Serve immediately or let sit in the fridge for 3-5 minutes, covering with food wrap.
Gods' nectar!

Chia Pudding

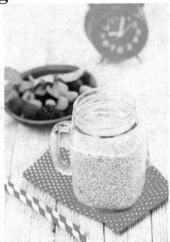

Ingredients:
- ½ cup coconut milk
- 1 tbsp Chia seeds
- 3 tbsp coconut water
- 1 tsp vanilla extract
- ½ tsp cinnamon

Nutrition 100 g:
Calories: 284 kcal
Carbs: 5 g
Proteins: 5 g
Fat: 26 g

Directions:
1. In a glass bowl, mix coconut milk, coconut water, Chia seeds.
2. Add the vanilla extract and cinnamon.
3. Mix everything well.
4. Cover with food wrap, refrigerate to gel (minimum 1.5 hours, maximum 1 night).
5. Serve cold and garnish with red berries, brittle or other.
Wellness made pudding!

The Princess's Cake

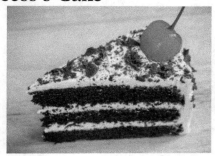

Ingredients:
Base:

- 1 egg yolk and 1 whipped egg white
- ¼ cup almond flour - 1 tbsp coconut flour
- 1 tsp psyllium
- 50 g Dark chocolate (80%), without sugars
- 3 tbsp clarified butter
- ¼ sachet of Bertolini vanilla yeast
- ½ tsp vanilla- 2 tbsp erythritol

Filling:

- 1 cup fresh cream- 1 tsp erythritol
- 20 gr dark chocolate (8%), without sugars
- 1 tbsp cherry jam light

Nutrition 100 g:
Calories: 374 kcal **Carbs:** 5 g **Proteins:** 20 g **Fat:** 26 g
Directions:
1. Whisk yolk and erythritol in a large bowl. Add all other ingredients and incorporate beaten egg whites.
3. Pour into a buttered 4 inches mold and bake at 360° F for 30 minutes. Allow cooling completely before cutting into 3 discs for filling.
5. Whip the cream and add the sweeteners when the cream is already almost fully whipped.
6. Stuff the discs and stack. Cover with cream on top and around. Sprinkle with grated chocolate on top and around.
7. Garnish on top with tufts of whipped cream and decorate with tiny tufts of jam (or sugar-free natural cherries in syrup). Refrigerate. Serve cold. You'll feel like eating a cake in a castle!